fighting
globesity

fighting globesity

Phillip and Jackie Mills, M.D.

RANDOM HOUSE
NEW ZEALAND

A catalogue record for this book is available from the National Library of New Zealand.

A RANDOM HOUSE BOOK
published by
Random House New Zealand
18 Poland Road, Glenfield, Auckland, New Zealand
www.randomhouse.co.nz

Random House International
Random House
20 Vauxhall Bridge Road
London, SW1V 2SA
United Kingdom

Random House Australia (Pty) Ltd
20 Alfred Street, Milsons Point, Sydney,
New South Wales 2061, Australia

Random House South Africa Pty Ltd
Isle of Houghton
Corner Boundary Road and Carse O'Gowrie
Houghton 2198, South Africa

Random House Publishers India Private Ltd
301 World Trade Tower, Hotel Intercontinental Grand Complex,
Barakhamba Lane, New Delhi 110 001, India

First published 2007

© 2007 Phillip and Jackie Mills

ISBN 978 1 86941 854 0

Design: Nic Hall
Layout: Anna Seabrook
Cover and internal illustrations: gettyimages
Cover design: Nic Hall
Printed in Australia by Griffin Press

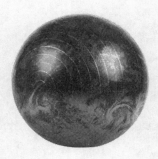

contents

For Diana and Les

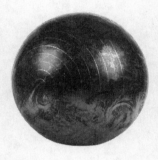

introduction | important — read this first

Globesity is a term we use to describe the relationship that currently operates between personal fitness, national health systems and global sustainability.

We believe it's an important relationship, and that if you understand it you'll be empowered and motivated to take some simple actions, *essential* actions, that will dramatically improve your life and make a powerful contribution to the health of our planet.

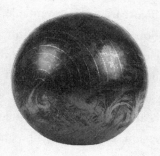

what the hell is globesity?

So what the hell is globesity and how does the relationship work?

Globesity begins in our own back yard. People in the developed world are getting busier and busier. We now work 30 per cent more hours than we did in the 1960s. We no longer have time for traditional sports and leisure activities. We don't exercise, we eat calorie-rich fast food and consequently we get fat — *really* fat.

Over 30 per cent of Americans are now clinically obese and 70 per cent — *70 per cent* — are either overweight or obese. Three hundred thousand people a year die from obesity-related diseases in the US alone.

And it's not just an American problem: the rest of the world is catching up fast. Obesity levels in most developed nations have doubled during the past two decades. In New Zealand, traditionally regarded as sporting and healthy, adult obesity rates almost doubled between 1989 and 2003 to 21 per cent.

Obesity is currently overtaking cigarette smoking as the number one killer in developed nations and is predicted to take yet another exponential leap as the current generation gets older.

In families these days, it's the norm for both parents to work. We don't have the time to take our kids to play sports and we don't have the time — or in some cases the knowledge — to give them the right food. So our kids play computer games and eat junk food and they get fat too.

This is the first generation in which widespread childhood obesity has occurred and it's spreading at an alarming rate, even in the developing nations of Asia and Latin America. Our generation of parents may be the first in history to watch our children die before us — of preventable, known illnesses.

Obesity has become a global pandemic, the burden of which can be a real hell for those who are a part of it. Aside from the millions worldwide who are dying early, there are now more than a billion of us whose quality of life is diminished by overweight- or inactivity-related illnesses such as type 2 diabetes, many cancers, heart disease, strokes, osteoporosis, inflammation, immune deficiency, depression, cognitive decline and dementia. But this is just a part of the globesity picture . . .

The weight of the problem

A series of front-page features in *The New York Times* in January 2006 noted that some New York suburbs have overweight-related type 2 diabetes rates as high as 50 per cent! Type 2 diabetes, which is just one obesity-driven disease, is estimated to have cost the US economy US$130 billion in 2006 — more than the entire Gross Domestic Product (GDP) of New Zealand! *The New York Times* series quoted senior health officials and hospital managers saying that at present rates of growth, the already overburdened American hospital system would collapse under the weight of this epidemic (their pun, not ours). And a 2006 *British Medical Journal* report warned that rising levels of obesity in the UK could bankrupt the National Health Service if left unchecked.

The cost of the American health system, like many others, is already spiralling out of control. In 2006 it was an estimated $2.1 trillion, accounting for approximately 17 per cent of US GDP and costing $7000 for every man, woman and child in the country. In each of the seven years prior to that, it grew by around 10 per cent, compared with 2 per cent inflation.

You may have heard the quip that General Motors is no longer in the automobile business; it's a health insurance company that makes cars to support its habit. In 2004 GM's healthcare schemes cost $5.1 billion — almost $5000 per employee — and added $1500 to the cost of every one of its cars.

Seventy-five per cent of US health costs are spent on the treatment of chronic illness, a large proportion of which stems directly from *inactivity* among the aged and the overweight.

Seen from this perspective, the obesity epidemic presents a crisis that is disastrous not only for those suffering directly from it, but for everyone else as well. However, to see the whole globesity picture we need to take a further step back and consider it in the context of even bigger trends . . .

The big (fat) picture

Consider these statistics: members of First World economies — roughly 20 per cent of the world's population — currently consume approximately 80 per cent of the world's annual resource production. At present levels of human efficiency and technology, this level of consumption is unsustainable. We are running out of natural resources, from fossil oil to farmable land, from fish in our oceans to the water we drink.

Assuming we don't reach a disastrous tipping point with global warming over the next 10–20 years, we could probably deal with these issues through a modest effort from government, business and individuals . . . if everything else remained equal. The problem is that everything else will not remain equal. Over the next 50 years world population is likely to grow by 50 per cent to 9.5 billion and it is predicted that *half* of the current non-First World population will move to First World consumer status.

The World Wildlife Fund's 'Living Planet Report', released in October 2006, states that in 2003 we were outstripping the Earth's capacity to regenerate resources by 25 per cent; unless there is a dramatic and immediate change in consumption patterns, within 50 years the world's population will use 200 per cent more resources than the planet can produce.

If we don't change, we face the unfortunate irony of the current obesity epidemic being replaced by one of starvation. For six of the last seven years the world has produced less food than we have all eaten and we have been munching into stockpiles to make up the difference. As a result the stockpiles have dropped from being sufficient to feed everyone on Earth for 116 days in 1999 to sufficient for only 57 days in 2006, the lowest for more than 30 years.

Like an overweight individual, as a race we are simply consuming far more than we can healthily maintain. And we have started to discover the 'inconvenient truth' (to use Al Gore's phrase) that some of the resulting illnesses — atmospheric destruction, resource-based wars and economic disasters, for instance — cannot be insulated against by class barriers or national borders. In today's globalised world these things affect us all. We *all*, therefore, have a huge challenge ahead to create global sustainability.

Becoming part of the solution

There's a future out there that's way worth fighting for. The past 100 years have seen incredible advances for humanity. There's been a revolution in democracy and human rights. Technology is making knowledge and education available to all. Many of the major diseases have been conquered. We have the real ability to make poverty and hunger history.

If we can face the ecological challenges of the next 50 years, Planet Earth could be a pretty cool place to be in the future. To succeed in facing those challenges, governments, businesses and individuals all have a part to play. Some of the main things we need to do are:

- Move a *lot* more quickly to reduce our dependence on oil as an energy source — not only to reduce carbon dioxide (CO_2) emissions, but also to avert oil-price-based economic disasters and to remove the incentive for conflict in oil-producing areas.

  Part of this battle is being fought on a vast international stage between governments and huge, vested-interest corporations, who just don't seem to get the fact that *there's no more business if there's no more human civilisation.*

  On the positive side, pro-sustainability government is gaining momentum and the smart money in business is starting to side with the environment — whether altruistically or to make a buck. On the negative side, the bad guys have more money. However, individuals en masse can make this battle a no-contest by switching to green energy suppliers, installing solar energy systems in our homes, driving hybrid cars (better still, riding bikes), promoting workplace energy audits and many other ways we'll talk about in Parts Two and Three of this book.

- Support the growing sustainable farming movement — the shift to food production methods that preserve water, topsoil, soil fertility, marine and other wild food sources, and minimise deforestation, pollution and production of greenhouse gases. As we'll describe in Part Two, eating organic foods and de-polluting our environment will not only do a huge amount of good for our personal health, but also help preserve the planet.

- Push for methods of construction, manufacturing, distribution and raw material extraction that maximise energy efficiency and minimise waste and pollution. Things like the green architecture movement, recycling programmes and campaigns against packaging are essential to our future survival. Part Three outlines some simple ways to support them.

- Finally, it's clear that we face a titanic struggle in dealing with the above challenges. Adding burdens like those resulting from inactivity and overconsumption is a luxury we can no longer afford. Societies must choose where they allocate their scarce resources (in economic terms, make 'guns or butter' choices); money spent supporting overburdened health systems cannot be directed toward saving the planet.

Fitness is a sustainability issue

If we can start to win the battle against obesity and inactive ageing, then many of the *trillions* of dollars spent on chronic illness can be diverted to more important endeavours like protecting rainforests and subsidising sustainable energy programmes. And as it turns out, many of the actions involved in winning that battle — such as walking and riding bikes, or eating healthier, less fattening food — contribute symbiotically to solving our planet's larger problems.

Dealing with this is the main purpose of this book: to tackle globesity, starting with your very own battle for health, fitness and well-being. While we deal with the larger ecological issues in Part Three, the whole of Part One is devoted simply to the most powerful strategies we know for getting yourself enjoyably active; Part Two presents dietary tactics for weight loss and for improving your health. We'll show you how, starting in our own back yards, we can all make a huge contribution to global sustainability in ways that can also improve our lives and be a lot of fun.

Growing awareness

We've been concerned about the worsening health of society for some time. The mission of our companies has long been to improve people's lives. But like most concerned citizens, we've started to get alarmed about the bigger picture more recently.

The consequences of global warming are becoming obvious, even to the most intransigent of sceptics. Al Gore's documentary *An Inconvenient Truth* opened many eyes to this problem, and books like *Heat* by George Monbiot and *The Weathermakers* by Tim Flannery go a step further in spelling out the issue.

Scientists like Flannery and Jared Diamond have also brought the challenges to broader sustainability into the spotlight through their books *Collapse* (Diamond), and *The Future Eaters* and *The Eternal Frontier* (Flannery).

On a more personal scale, we were motivated to become part of the solution by the death of Phillip's mother. Colleen Mills was as healthy as a person could be. She played sport all her life and was still running masters track and field well into her 60s. She always ate healthily and was slim and very fit. Everyone thought she would live to be 120. Colleen was a hugely productive person in society, using her energies to good purpose. She worked with charities, acted in sports administration, organised women's groups; she helped a lot of people and died far too young at 71. Ironically, her pursuit of a healthy life was what killed her.

New Zealand is one of the cleanest, greenest countries in the world, but we're disproportionately inheriting one of the consequences of humanity's environmental sins. The hole in the ozone layer above Antarctica drifts over our country and southeastern Australia during the summer months and occasionally at other times of the year. Extended exposure to our sun causes serious skin damage, and Auckland and Sydney have had the distinction of being the melanoma capitals of the world for decades.

Phillip's mother died of skin cancer. She spent too much time outside in the sun, training for her beloved sport. She was first told that she had terminal melanoma in 2003 and she died in 2005. There is a direct link between our abuse of the environment and melanoma.

When chlorofluorocarbons (CFCs) were first introduced in the 1930s they were welcomed as a boon for society. They were a safe alternative to toxic, early-generation refrigeration chemicals, which could be fatal if they leaked. These had, in turn, replaced the necessity to cart blocks of ice around neighbourhoods.

In the mid-1970s scientists identified the possibility that CFCs could destroy ozone in the upper atmosphere, but it was not until the discovery of a huge hole in the ozone layer above Antarctica in 1984 that moves began to phase out these compounds. It took until 1990 and massive international regulation in the form of the Montreal Protocol for the corporate chemical giants to stop manufacturing CFCs in the US and other developed countries. Under the terms of the protocol, production was allowed to continue in the Third World until 2010 and it will take an estimated 50–100 years for the ozone layer to be fully restored.

However, the good news is that the Montreal Protocol was signed and ozone levels appear at this stage to have stabilised. Despite the fact that the Third World was able to continue production under the treaty, production there slowed much more quickly than expected when the rest of the world switched technologies. And despite lobbying about the financial disasters the legislation would bring, the net result appears to have been an actual increase in economic productivity, stemming from the new industries created around CFCs' replacements.

By comparison, it is estimated that if the protocol hadn't been adopted, we'd now have 30 per cent less ozone, and the resulting bombardment of radiation would be causing a cataclysmic increase in human and animal cancers and crop destruction.

Does that scenario sound familiar? The debate around the Montreal Protocol was a smaller-scale version of what's now occurring with global warming. We've known for decades that activities such as the burning of fossil fuels cause carbon dioxide and other greenhouse gases to build up, trapping solar rays and heating up the atmosphere. In 1997, there was sufficient scientific concern that countries around the world signed the Kyoto Protocol, which committed industrialised nations to reducing carbon emissions to five per cent below 1990 levels by 2010 (29 per cent lower than what was otherwise predicted).

Since then, carbon emissions have continued to rise. The government of the United States, the world's biggest producer of CO_2 (by almost double the rate of all Europe combined), signed but has refused to ratify the protocol. China and India, who are exempt under the protocol as developing nations, have industrialised rapidly, to the point that they are challenging the US and a slowly decreasing Europe for first and third places on the ladder of major greenhouse gas producers. An overwhelming majority of the world's experts agree that even if successful, the Kyoto Protocol will be nowhere near enough to solve the problem. It must be superseded by a much more far-reaching version that needs to be enacted sooner than planned.

The effects of global warming are much bigger and more potentially catastrophic than those of ozone depletion. The well-publicised Stern Report, a 2006 study for the British finance ministry led by former World Bank chief economist Sir Nicholas Stern, says that a failure to immediately address greenhouse gas emissions will cost the world trillions of dollars, causing a catastrophic global recession and creating hundreds of millions of refugees — the largest migration in human history. The longer we delay dramatic action, the study says, the more it will cost us in the future.

At the extreme end, if we should reach a major tipping point like the collapse of the Amazon or the cessation of the Gulf Stream, the potential for major climate shifts increases to truly frightening levels, with consequences that will take not hundreds but thousands of years to repair and will result in the destruction of most existing life on Earth (as has occurred several times in our planet's history).

What we can do

Solving the problem of global warming will involve responsible acts of government on a scale never seen before. There is a need for massive regulation and cross-border co-operation based on putting aside selfish national agendas. It is no longer possible for industrialised nations to say that we will not participate in international agreements until developing nations are similarly bound. Only proactive policies will give us a chance of success.

Nor is it possible to say that I, or my company, will not contribute — that we will leave the responsibility to our neighbours. Rapid, decisive action needs to be taken by an overwhelming majority of businesses and individuals.

Only generosity in this case will ensure a desirable future for our children and grandchildren.

To those concerned about the potential costs, it's worth noting that many independent business experts believe that, as with the Montreal Protocol, there will be positive economic opportunities we cannot currently anticipate. But whether this is the case or not, the risk of the alternative is unthinkable. As parents *and* as business people, we can't imagine why any sane person would be prepared to take that risk.

To those already taking action on global warming, you have our admiration and respect. But we can't afford to rest on our laurels. Remember, climate change is just one of the sustainability challenges we face.

For many of us, on a personal level our sustainability challenge begins with the health of the place we live — our bodies.

Most of the actions we can take to meet these challenges, both personal and global, will improve our health, be fun, and enrich our lives in all sorts of ways. We know that you will reap rewards on so many levels when you get started on your own crusade. Whether it's throwing away the car keys and riding your bike to work, eating sustainable-organic foods, joining a walking group, or any of the other choices we talk about in this book, you'll feel better and your life will be much improved. Each one of us can make a difference. This book is full of practical steps we can take. Right now. Not tomorrow or when we find more time. Right now. The world can't wait.

About us

phillip   I was born in Auckland, New Zealand in 1955. My parents, Les and Colleen, were both athletes and my earliest childhood memories are of watching them and their friends training and competing in track and field events. Les competed at four Olympic Games in the shotput and discus, and Colleen was a New Zealand representative in the Commonwealth Games

400 m event when she was 41. Our family home overlooked Western Suburbs Athletic Club, which in those days was New Zealand's leading track and field venue. I can remember seeing legendary milers Peter Snell and Kip Keino race on the track below.

When I was seven, we moved to California so that my father could pursue his athletics career and his business studies. He studied at, and competed for, the University of Southern California. During this time my sister and I went to 32nd Street School in downtown LA. It was both literally and figuratively a world away from Grey Lynn Primary School in New Zealand.

Throughout my teens, attending Mt Albert Grammar School back in New Zealand, I was obsessed with two loves — music and sport. My father's prominence in athletics (he served for a number of years as New Zealand National Director of Track and Field Coaching) meant that I had the good fortune to be tutored and mentored by some of history's leading coaches, including Arthur Lydiard and US legend Tom Tellez. I was lucky enough to go to UCLA on a track scholarship and I graduated with a BA in Philosophy in 1978.

Music had always been a passion of mine and after I graduated I managed a well-known New Zealand rock band who had moved to LA for 18 months in 1978–79. I didn't realise it at the time, but the two interests that had consumed me as a teenager and into my early 20s were about to collide spectacularly.

My parents had always been involved in weight lifting as part of their training. In fact, half of our original family home was the gym for the Auckland Weightlifting Federation. In 1968 they opened their first commercial gym, Les Mills World of Fitness, and both had hands-on involvement — designing training programmes for members and overseeing every aspect of the club.

That club has played a significant role in the evolution of the global fitness industry. During the 80s it gained a cult reputation as host to the world's biggest aerobics sessions, with nightly attendances of up to 300 people per class. Since the mid-90s it has become known throughout the industry as the home of BodyPump™ and other branded Les Mills classes that are licensed by more than 11,000 gyms around the world. It currently has 12,000 members, with 7500 participants per week attending fitness classes, and it is visited every year by hundreds of overseas club owners and instructors.

While I was in LA in the late 70s I saw the start of the worldwide aerobics movement. It was the beginning of a global revolution in the way that people, especially women, exercised. I came back to New Zealand full of enthusiasm for this new fitness activity and convinced my parents that the aerobics craze was really going to be something special. I recruited friends from the sports and entertainment communities and travelled throughout New Zealand and Australia, publicising aerobics, training instructors and opening fitness clubs. It was at the new Les Mills club in Dunedin that I met Jackie. Wow!

After floating one of the world's first publicly listed fitness companies in 1984, my parents eventually sold their interests in the Les Mills World of Fitness clubs (later I set about buying the clubs back). Dad went on to serve three terms as mayor of Auckland City and Mum was fully involved in community affairs right up to her death in 2005.

Since 1990, Jackie and I, along with our two children Diana and Les, have been on a wild ride. We created BodyPump, a barbell class aimed at making weight lifting more fun, and the world went crazy for it. Seventy thousand instructors now teach BodyPump and other branded Les Mills programmes, and every week more than five million people do a Les Mills class in 73 countries around the world.

We have been very fortunate to receive some rewards and awards along the way. In 2004 I was named as New Zealand's Ernst & Young Entrepreneur of the Year and, having been a finalist at the world awards in Monte Carlo, I was invited to return as a judge in 2006.

These experiences have had a profound effect on my world view.

My interest in holistic nutrition and sustainable farming has been honed both by Jackie and by my sister Donna, a long-term specialist in the field, who has recently opened a 40 hectare state-of-the-art teaching centre at Omori Bay, Lake Taupo, showcasing environmental sustainability.

jackie | When I first met Phillip I knew that going on the road with him would be something pretty cool — and so it has been.

I was born in Te Awamutu, a small town in the North Island. My dad, Peter Bull, was one of New Zealand's leading school principals and so we moved a bit when I was growing up. Dad was always playing sport; he was a provincial rugby representative and played competitive cricket into his 60s. My sisters and brother and I were fully immersed in exercise as the way to spend any spare time. As a teenager I represented New Zealand in gymnastics under the awesome coach Emmy Bellwood and travelled through Europe with the national team. After high school I went to Otago University for four years and graduated with a Physical Education degree. It was there that I met Phillip and the next few years were a whirlwind of travel throughout Australasia as we spread the word about aerobics. I loved being super-fit and healthy, and the buzz of aerobics was completely addictive.

In 1984, when we returned to New Zealand, I wanted to understand more about health and well-being, so I started a medical degree at Auckland University. During my work on my degree we were blessed with two wonderful children. I'm enormously grateful for the support of family and friends who helped me balance the demands of study, work and raising Diana and Les.

Exercise has always been such a vital part of my life. In 1991 I went to the Aerobics World Cup in Tokyo and finished seventh, and I've kept up a schedule of teaching aerobics classes, competitive running and other sports.

As my interest in women's health grew, I completed a Diploma in Obstetrics and Gynaecology and began working alongside an 'alternative' general practitioner, the late John Hilton. At times I was helping as many as 30 women birth per month, many of those in the women's own homes. It was a busy time but interest in the alternative approaches to birth and women's health we offered meant that demand for our services was high. Sadly, choices for women have decreased as government policy changes have made it unviable for GPs to continue to deliver babies, and I finally stopped practising obstetrics in 2003.

I'm still working part time as a doctor at a holistic center in Point Chevalier in Auckland. I chose this environment because I have always been disillusioned with traditional medicine, where doctors are often forced to see a different patient every ten minutes and prescribe drugs rather than having the time to uncover the root causes of illness. I now focus on nutritional medicine, exercise, counselling and alternative therapies. I still prescribe drugs, but only as a last resort. This approach has been phenomenal — I've witnessed at first hand the dramatic changes in a person's health when nutritional, exercise and psychological needs are addressed. Long-term illnesses can disappear and patients' lives are transformed.

I also work as a creative director for Les Mills International and head the BodyBalance™ programme — known in the US as BodyFlow™. This class combines yoga, t'ai chi and Pilates and is designed to reduce stress, increase flexibility, and restore mind/body harmony and balance. Diana has left home now and Les will soon head off to an American university to play basketball. This has given me that little bit of extra time to pause and reflect on our life journey so far. I love nearly everything about what I do (we could all do with less paperwork — right?) and am happy to have this opportunity to share some of the lessons we've taken from the last 25 years.**)**

Fighting globesity

The book is divided into three parts. Part One deals with the most effective, successful ways to create an exercise-based lifestyle. There are four key elements to this and each is presented in its own chapter.

The first, Become Some Body, deals with motivating yourself, goal setting and creating lifelong habits. Chapter 2, Forever Fitness, is about making fitness part of your social schedule — a habit-building system that will enrich your life. Chapter 3, It's A Game Of Inches, talks about the best ways to make exercise *fun*. Chapter 4, Free The Mind, The Body will Follow, explains some of the science and shows you the fastest, most efficient techniques to get results from your efforts.

At its most basic, getting into shape is built on two things: the energy you put out and the energy you put in. Part One focuses on the 'energy out' side of the equation and Part Two on 'energy in'. In Chapter 5, Downsize Me, we summarise the most proven, successful methods for controlling your calorie intake and provide a few new ones of our own. Chapter 6, Shape Your World, is about how to eat more nutritious, less-polluted food, the growing popularity of which is important not only for improving our health, but also in solving our ecological problems. In Chapter 7, Eat Your Medicine, we present cutting-edge ways in which food and careful, targeted supplementation can be used to cure many medical conditions.

Part Three moves from personal to global health. Chapters 8 to 12 are an overview of the broader environmental problems we face. Chapter 13, It Comes From In Here, is a summary of actions, beyond exercising more and eating better, that we can all take to help us successfully face the major sustainability-related challenges ahead.

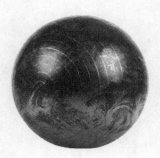

part one | energy out

Sustainability starts with your own body. If we can start to win the battle against obesity and inactive ageing, then many of the *trillions* of dollars spent on chronic illness can be diverted into more important endeavours such as saving rainforests and subsidising sustainable energy programmes. The first part of this book is devoted simply to explaining the most powerful strategies we know for getting yourself enjoyably active.

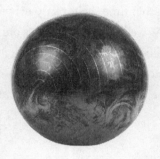

1 | become some body

On your marks, get set, go!

phillip

When my mother, Colleen, was in her late 30s, she wanted to start exercising again. She was very out of shape. As a teenager she had played basketball and competed in athletics, but then she married, had children and worked hard for 20 years raising us and building the family business. As we started to get more independent she wanted to establish a life for herself again. My sister Donna and I were training for track and field then, so Mum decided she would do that too. She came to the Western Suburbs club at Grey Lynn Park, where we used to train, and she couldn't jog even a single 400 m lap of the track. She was so unfit, she could jog for about 50 m and then she'd have to stop and walk the rest of the way.

But bit by bit, she built herself up. She came along with us each week and gradually she would walk less and run more, until she found she could jog a lap without stopping. Then she could jog two laps, then she could jog a mile and eventually, over time, she built up to the point where she started doing sprint training and actually competitively running the 400 m. She could run 10 km as part of her training programme and she could do tough interval workouts on the track. In 1974, she won a New Zealand title in the 400 m. That year she made the Commonwealth Games team, representing New Zealand in the 400 m. She was 41.

It took her about four years to get to that point. She went on to compete in masters track and field meets, and became world champion in numerous events. She competed at that level well into her 60s. She got so much joy out of competing again. During that time she took up teaching aerobics and did that through to her late 50s. As well, she got all of her old girlfriends together, and they played indoor basketball well into their 60s.

My mother had developed a whole new life: a completely out-of-shape person who couldn't jog one lap of a track became somebody who was inspirational.

STRATEGY 1 | TAKE UP A SPORT

Nothing will motivate you as powerfully to exercise. Whether it's training for a 10 km run, a tennis tournament or a rock and roll dancing competition, fix your eyes on the prize and go for it. Once people get hooked into a sport, they forget about having to motivate themselves and actually start to look forward to their next training session. They get excited about the chance it provides to improve, to move closer to their goals. The exercise becomes secondary to the passion of taking part, improving and learning new skills. The next thing you know you're looking in the mirror and hey, there's an athlete's body looking back!

We'll talk more in Chapter 3 about some of the options available (including many which are non-competitive) and how to choose between them, but for a start try the following: anything you did when you were younger, anything your friends are doing, anything that has a club nearby or anything that gives you a thrill.

BHAGS — set yourself a ridiculous goal

Once you've started, the most powerful thing you can do is set yourself a major goal within your chosen sport. Many people exercise because they have to (or want to) lose weight. That might be a big enough goal in itself: if your doctor has said you've got to get your blood pressure down or you'll die, that is a powerful motivation! But we *really* don't want it to get that serious.

We believe that everyone should set major fitness goals: powerful aims that create a much more holistic impetus to exercise. People in business these days call them BHAGs — Big Hairy Audacious Goals — a term originally coined by Jim Collins, author of the business classic *Good To Great*.

It's something that anybody can do, whether you're preparing for a bike race, training with an adult swim group or working out at the gym. Depending on your start point, it might be anything from competing in a national championship in your chosen sport to finishing in the top 1000 in the New York Marathon.

There's a power in allowing yourself to dream, in visualising yourself at your very best. It can be incredibly inspiring and motivating. Great coaches often use this technique very effectively.

I've mentioned that as a teenager I was lucky enough to train occasionally with Arthur Lydiard. Arthur was the coach credited by Nike co-founder Bill Bowerman and many others as fathering the modern jogging boom.

In the 1960s and 70s, New Zealand, with a population at the time of just 2.5 million, dominated the world in distance running. We had Olympic champions Peter Snell in the 800 and the 1500 m, Murray Halberg in the 5000 m, and John Walker in the 1500 m. We had Dick Quax, Olympic silver medallist and world-record holder at 5000 m, Olympic medallists Barry McGee and Mike Ryan in the marathon, and Rod Dixon and John Davies in the 1500 m. Arthur coached most of these athletes, or inspired their coaches. He was later headhunted as national coach for Finland, which, along with Kenya, came to rival New Zealand as a world leader of the sport during the 70s.

Arthur could give you a dream, a vision of yourself at your best. He would convince you that it was possible for you to win an Olympic gold medal. He would just say matter of factly, 'Well, if you do this and this and this, you can win the Olympics.'

I remember my father telling me about rooming with Peter Snell at the 1960 Olympics and asking him how he thought he would do in the 800 m. As a 19 year old who had barely qualified for the games, Snell replied: 'Well, Arthur says I've done the preparation to win it . . . I think I can win it.' He did just that, shocking the world by beating the world-record holder, Roger Moens.

Of course, not everybody can win an Olympic gold medal, but having that dream, having that vision, inspires you to train really hard and get the best out of yourself.

That's the thing about BHAGs. If you set an easy goal, then you won't train as hard: the higher the target you set, the harder you have to try, the more you have to streamline everything that you do in your training to be effective. Even if you don't make it, you'll get further than you ever would have without an audacious goal.

I always set big goals and big visions for myself when I was competing in athletics. The Olympic dream was something that powerfully inspired and motivated me.

In the end, I never did win an Olympic gold medal. In fact, I didn't even get to compete in an Olympic Games. I qualified six times for Montreal in 1976 and the bronze medal went just 0.2 sec outside my best, but as I was a student residing in the United States I wasn't selected for the New Zealand team.

But although I failed to achieve my big goal, my years of being involved in sport were an incredible experience. I had an international competitive career where I got to combine study and training and compete in athletics all over the world. I still look back on that time as one of the best parts of my life. I didn't win an Olympic medal, but I got to the point of not being bad at the 400 m hurdles and I had some amazing experiences.

I had the great joy of competition, the pleasure of feeling my body at its absolute peak, and I met many wonderful people who have remained lifelong friends.

Trust me, I've been there

Later on in my life I went through a more difficult period. In 1987, our family's publicly listed company was bought out but I stayed on as manager. About a month after that, the 1987 sharemarket crash occurred and the companies that had taken over our company went into receivership. So I embarked on a campaign to buy it back. I had to borrow heavily to do this and I had to commit myself to years of hard work to pay off the loans. About the same time, we had our children: Diana was born in 1986, followed by Les in 1988. I'd taken on this tremendous test, so I ended up going through a very hard work phase of my life.

Five years later, I came out the other end of that tunnel, absolutely burned out. I was way out of shape and had put on ten kg. For someone like me, this was hard. I'd competed in athletics throughout the 70s, I'd taught fitness classes through to 1987, and then I'd done nothing at all for about five years. I was suffering from mild depression.

I talked to Jackie about it and she said: 'Well, let's set some goals.' I thought, 'Okay, what kind of goals can I set?' I wanted to establish a sporting goal that would suit our lifestyle. We still had young kids, so I didn't want to choose a sport that was going to take me away from home a lot. I'd played a bit of tennis at high school, so that was something that I felt I could do. I'm not one to do anything by halves, so with Jackie's support we knocked down our garage and took out half of our yard and managed to squeeze a tennis court in beside the house. Then I set myself this ridiculous goal of playing national-level tennis. I had no idea what that really entailed and if I had told anybody who did, they would have laughed at me. But that was just the way I thought about it.

I knew I couldn't do it on my own: I'd need some help. So I started with a coach and found some guys who were willing to play with me. Twice a week I'd have the coach, then every weekend we'd have a big game where the guys would come around and we'd play for about three hours. I don't know how I ever thought I was going to play top-level tennis by training three times a week, but gradually over time I improved. I increased the number of weekly sessions and games to five, and actually started to learn the game, which meant I was able to properly enjoy the tactical and mental aspects of it as well as the physical challenge.

Of course, I never got anywhere near playing at a national level. I pretty quickly set more realistic 'interim' goals. But over the next five years I got to the point where I could play at a decent B-grade level and I could play in competitions. I got good enough that I could travel overseas with friends to play in pro-am tennis tournaments like the Fiji Open.

I had a few mates who were really good national-level players, such as Craig

Hansford, Gary Oliver and my coach Bruce Derlin, who'd been ranked in the top 100 on the ATP circuit. They would come over some weekends and play in our three-hour Sunday doubles games. I got such excitement, exhilaration and joy from just being on the court with guys who could play tennis at that level.

Throughout this process, of course, my need for exercise became incidental as my goals and passion for the game took over. But in the process I lost 7 kg. And I lost my depression in a matter of weeks! I firmly believe that just by setting the goal and starting to exercise again I was able to radically alter my state of mind and sense of well-being. (We document some of the research showing that exercise is a great first-line treatment for people with depression in Chapter 4.)

Setting that big goal motivated me to establish a regular training routine and to start enjoying my life again. And I know that I was a better father and husband, too, because I felt as though I was getting back to a natural state of being: fit and healthy.

STRATEGY 2 SET YOURSELF A RIDICULOUS GOAL

Dream huge. Create a vision that will inspire and motivate you. The bigger the challenge, the more you will push yourself to a level that will take you to your absolute best.

Don't worry if you don't make it. At the start, you don't realise how good you have to be. You don't realise how good these guys are. Every level that you go up, every level that you grow, every mountaintop that you reach, you see the peak of the next one. You often realise that the goal you set in the beginning is one that you're never going to be able to achieve, but you know that what you got out of the journey was incredible fun.

Create a road map

When you start from scratch, set a baseline. If you're running, choose a pleasant scenic route and time your first outing. Go easy on yourself. Walk a little, jog a little. If you're swimming, it might be as many laps as you can comfortably do and you should make a note of the time. If you're counting steps on a pocket pedometer, do a manageable number. If you're lifting weights, start light and easy. For cycling, choose an agreeable route and take it at a leisurely pace. Don't try to bust a gut: this has to be natural and comfortable for you. You never want to create too much pain — that tends to build a psychological aversion to the activity, which can make you want to quit.

The next few times you may just repeat what you did the first time, or even make it a bit easier if it was tough. But after just two or three sessions you'll start to feel a natural urge to jog a little bit more and to walk a little bit less. Or you're going to swim a bit further, or a bit faster. At first you're going to do this three times a week, maybe later you'll want to take it to five. This becomes the basis of a training programme.

If your Tuesday run/walk took half an hour this week, then next week you're going to do that same route and do it half a minute faster. The week after that, another half a minute faster — and so on for six to twelve weeks, building up in small, achievable increments.

If your Thursday walk/run was 2 km this week, then next week you might increase it to 2.5 km, then 3, 3.5 etc. You'll eventually get to the point where you can comfortably go for 10 km.

Saturday might just be an hour-long scenic walk at quite a leisurely pace. Over the weeks you'll walk a bit faster and a bit further, and maybe start to throw in some jogging spells. You might get to the point where you're putting in an hour-long run, or an hour-long run/walk, depending on what you can handle.

To prevent yourself from getting bored, every 6–12 weeks you'll need to change the courses, speeds and distances, to mix it up.

This is the principle of setting yourself a training programme. It's simple. The conditioning part doesn't require an expert coach and it's the same for all sports. Whether it's running, cycling, swimming, weight-training or any other basic fitness activity, it's just a matter of setting yourself small, incremental targets, slightly faster times, slightly longer distances, slightly increased resistances etc and varying it all over time. Let your body evolve in the small steps to which it naturally aspires — steps that you can handle and that you enjoy.

Of course you *do* need coaching for the technique component of most activities, and there are a few other crucial elements you need to build into your workouts to create long-term sustainability, like social support and *fun*. These are available from many sources, which we'll talk about in Chapters 2 and 3. But in the meantime let's look at the next few steps involved in developing a programme.

> If you don't know where you're going,
> then how are you going to get there?

You might say: I'm going to run a marathon — or I'm going to do something bigger, like get good enough to qualify for the New York Marathon* or one of the other famous events around the world. You really can succeed. Remember, my mother represented New Zealand at the age of 41, after not being able to jog a lap. Anything's possible. That becomes your three- to five-year goal.

Next, you put lots of interim steps and milestones between then and now. Give yourself structure with lots of small, attainable goals. The small weekly improvements in speed or distance etc that are described above will lead to small milestone achievements at the end of each 6–12 week training cycle. It might be that you can complete one of your standard training courses in a new time or it could be participating in a real race.

If you live in my city, Auckland, you might start out by entering the Round the Bays run. Your first time out, you could set yourself the goal of running the course in under 60 minutes. (This fun run, which began in 1972, is one of the oldest in the world and has approximately 70,000 participants. It's only 8.4 km long, but because of the numbers many competitors start well behind the line and run further than that.)

Develop a programme that you believe will get you to the stage of being ready to achieve that 60-minute goal over three to six months. You can supplement the principles I've described above by getting more information from the web. Large public events for sports these days often have websites with training schedules and guidelines for beginners.

After you've executed your training programme and competed in that

---

* Guaranteed NY Marathon qualifying times range from approximately three to four hours, depending on sex and age. Outside of that you can enter by lottery. Around half of US and a quarter of overseas applicants are accepted through the lottery system. Go to *www.nycmarathon.org* for details.

first event, you might set yourself a goal to run it faster next year, and in the meantime target some other fun-run events including, eventually, some half marathons. Set your sights on a series of interim events and objectives that lead up to your big goal, be that completing a full marathon race or qualifying for New York.

If you're simply training at the gym with the ultimate aim of looking like Jessica Alba or Brad Pitt, you could aim to become a group fitness teacher or a part-time personal trainer. Or — and it may seem like a crazy idea right now — there are thousands of people around the world competing in all sorts of age-group figure and fitness competitions. These provide a great, healthy motivation to maximise your workouts and could be your BHAG.

To achieve that, you should create a bunch of little training goals and programmes that move you successfully toward each new level. You have to break that BHAG down into manageable chunks: there's no point in simply trying to run the New York Marathon with no training. You need to build up to the big event.

Mental preparation

We've all heard the expression that the difference between really talented sportspeople and the men and women who go on to become world champions is in the top two inches. Mental preparation is a hugely important part of any training programme.

After you've worked out your ridiculous goal and a training schedule to get you there, set little targets for yourself every time you work out: they might be run times, calorie burns, steps on a pedometer or weight lifts. Remind yourself of these goals before every workout. Take time before you even begin to warm up to focus on the individual aims you have for that session. There is an incredible power in your subconscious.

When I was training full time, the night before a training session, last thing before I went to sleep, I liked to think about what my goals were, in terms of how fast I was going to run my 300 m repetitions, or how fast I was going to run a five or ten km run, or how much I was going to lift in my squats. I'd also like to think about it a little during the daytime, before I worked out. I found that this mental preparation would make a big difference to the results I achieved during the session. If I didn't do this and I came in mentally cold, I would do much worse than if I had prepared properly.

This is a fascinating area of psychology, with a number of possible explanations. Perhaps the most common is based around the biology of our brains. The theory goes something like this: the part of your brain that controls movement, co-ordination and spatial awareness is your right cerebral cortex. You can access that part of your brain through relaxation and visualisation. When you're in a relaxed state and you visualise yourself doing things well — performing co-ordinated movements with good technique, or running quickly — then it sticks.

There have been a number of studies in which, for example, one group of people physically practised a series of basketball shots for a period of time and another group just visualised the shots. At the end of the study, the people who simply visualised the shots had almost as high a percentage improvement as those who practised them.

Another important reason to psych up before each workout is that when you succeed at something, you get a psychological reward — a reinforcement of the activity — and this helps create positive habits. On the flip side, the opposite is true: if you fail, then it's dispiriting. We're programmed to love winning and every time we achieve these little goals we get positive reinforcement that we are on track and this helps cement our exercise habits.

STRATEGY 3 CREATE A ROAD MAP

Write down your plans and goals and record your daily results in a training diary. Plan out a training programme with realistic annual, quarterly, weekly and daily targets. Like anything else in life, the more you plan, the better the results. Don't worry if you don't hit all of your targets: plans should be flexible. At the end of every stage, stop and re-evaluate. If you didn't achieve your goals, ask yourself, 'What can I do better to achieve them next time?' If you did reach them, ask, 'What can I do to improve even further?'

If necessary, adjust the plan. Make your short-term goals achievable and long-term ones audacious.

● | **ONE OF THE PERSONAL TRAINERS AT OUR GYM IN DUNEDIN TOLD ME THIS STORY:**

Sally, a client of mine, needed to lose 10 kg. She was overweight and her knees were troubling her; she was having pain if she walked further than from her front door to her letterbox. But she couldn't get excited about all the training just for weight loss and she was bored on the cardio machines. So we set her the goal of walking the Dunedin half marathon. We struggled away together and of course eventually Sally completed the race and lost the weight. But the most powerful transformation took place in her role as a mother. Previously, she'd never been involved in her children's sports, but as her weight came off and her fitness increased she started helping out with her son's soccer team and was asked to become the assistant coach. Her son had massive gains in confidence and together they researched and prepared soccer drill sessions for his team. They formed a much stronger bond. Plus Sally was able to go on school camp as a parent helper — the camp involved a five-hour hike into the bush to sleep under the stars; something she would not have even considered to be in the realms of possibility the year before.

> Sally, a client of mine, needed to lose 10 kg. So we set her the goal of walking the Dunedin half marathon.

The importance of training cycles

In sports conditioning, we call the process of setting interim training programmes *periodisation*. We talk about creating mini cycles and macro cycles within your programme that develop your capacity to achieve your longer-term goals. There are always things that you can't do, and your body has to go through a physical evolution to reach goals beyond that barrier. It could take anywhere from six weeks to four years or more, depending on the level of the goal and your level of ability.

Your body evolves through a process called adaptation and progression. For example, the average beginner in the gym can double his or her strength within six to twelve weeks of starting out — you can literally double the amount of weight you can lift. After that, you start to plateau. Basically, you shock your body, give it something it's not used to and you get gigantic gains over that six- to twelve-week period. When your body adapts and you hit a plateau, you have to find a different way of shocking it. You give it a different set of challenges and make it adapt again. In the gym we call this 'shock to unblock'.

Over time, as your body evolves, you're able to handle more and more. Your cycles become more and more intense, the physical challenges ever greater. You often find that what you struggle to achieve as a beginner becomes simply a part of your daily warm up as you progress.

There has been a great deal of controversy over how far to go with this. At elite level, some coaches believe in taking their athletes into deep troughs throughout the cycles and only allowing them to freshen up or 'taper' once or twice per year. Others believe that '*quality* practice makes perfect' and that a degree of freshness must be maintained all year round.

Several famous coaches have had only one or two athletes who were physically capable of surviving their regimes. Those few genetic freaks created the coaches' fame, but at a cost to many who worked themselves into the ground and never fulfilled their potential. On the other hand, I've seen poorly performing, over-trained athletes dramatically improve their performances after being forced to rest by the 'misfortune' of a minor injury.

Current work being done with top rugby players and sailors in New Zealand, measuring key biochemical markers at different times of the training and recovery cycles, shows that there really are different strokes for different folks. Each athlete has completely different hormonal and other physiological reactions to various workouts. The easy-to-administer tests, developed by HortResearch, are likely to become widely available in the future so that you will be able to determine exactly the right workout regime for your body.

In the meantime, you and I have to proceed by judicious trial and error, following the coaching models that have achieved broadest success.

Learn from the best

Arthur Lydiard's method was based on his now famous foundation-building 100-mile-a-week cycle, transitioning to a lower mileage period with interval training at the track, and culminating in six weeks of getting 'fresh and sharp' with sprint training. Athletes would go through that cycle several times a year, building up to the northern and southern hemispheres' competitive seasons, or the track, road and cross-country seasons.

In the 1970s, the assistant coach of our track team at UCLA was Tom Tellez — arguably the greatest track and field coach ever. Tom went on to become head coach at the University of Houston for 23 years. He coached Olympic gold medallist sprinters Carl Lewis, Leroy Burrell, Mike Marsh, Joe DeLoach and Michele Finn-Burrell. He also coached many Olympic field event medallists including Dwight Stones and my old UCLA roommate, pole-vaulter Mike Tully. Tom was a technical perfectionist, as anyone who has ever watched Carl Lewis run 100 m will know. He worked with you until you had perfect technique in your event. But he also operated on the basis of making it fun. The training cycles that he developed for different times of the season had a lot of variety in them, so that in the wintertime, the guys would sometimes just play soccer or do drills like jumping over an obstacle course; some were for developing co-ordination and others event-specific, but more importantly the schedule wasn't burning us out mentally or physically. He used to say that *the most important day of your training cycle is your rest day.*

So you set yourself a workout programme that lasts for six to twelve weeks, and within that cycle you have weekly cycles. This is important. Within each cycle your body needs to recover from each different type of exercise: you can't just do the same thing every day, or you quickly start to over-train and you get diminishing returns. This is quite common, even at elite athlete level. Some people become so obsessively driven that they don't rest up and recover. They don't get the most out of themselves. They get injured, they get sick. They stop progressing properly and start to go downhill. Work out hard, and then rest.

Cross-training

One way to maximise your workouts is to challenge your body in different ways on successive days — both to avoid over-training and to develop different areas of your fitness. This is one reason why we *cross-train.*

Cross-training means varying the types of sports or activities we perform during a cycle. We allow one set of muscles or physiological system to rest, while exercising another. It's a way of maximising both the amount of work we can do in a week and the benefits of the different types of exercise. There are also synergies in combining certain activities; they produce benefits that complement each other.

For example, to develop speed you might do sprint training and technique drills at the track one day, then weight training at the gym the next. On the sprint training day you're developing reflex speed, technique, conditioning etc. But leg strength is an important part of speed and the most effective way to develop it is by doing exercises like leg squats in the gym. (Of course you can't just do squats; you have to do some other exercises to keep you balanced. For instance, you need to supplement the back work involved in squatting with some strengthening exercises for your abs or you'll wind up getting back pain; you may also need to do some hamstring exercises to balance the quadriceps strength created by the squats and avoid hamstring pulls.) By alternating the two activities day by day you not only cover all the bases in terms of the training requirements of your sport, but also allow your body to recover from one type of activity while working it out doing another.

Another good example of the benefits of cross-training is in working out for weight loss. Losing fat requires that you alter the balance of the energy in/energy out equation i.e. you expend more energy by exercising than you take in through your diet. To achieve this you'll need plenty of aerobic activity like running, cycling or swimming. But an essential part of any weight-loss programme is (and some people are surprised by this) strength training.

When we lift weights, we build the size of our muscle fibres — and that increases the size of our fat-burning engine. You don't have to look like the Incredible Hulk, just a small percentage gain will do. Every ounce of extra muscle fibre you carry exponentially increases the amount of energy you burn during your aerobic training.

In a 13-week study by the University of Auckland's sports science department for Les Mills in 1998, BodyPump — a weight-training class — had the lowest calorie-burning effect during the workout of all our fitness classes. But at the end of the study, Body Pump had *by far* the highest result of percentage body-fat loss.*

Variety is the spice of fitness

As I've said, you might typically do a particular type of exercise for six to twelve weeks. Partly, this will be determined by when you start to hit your plateau. As soon as you start to hit a plateau and you stop improving at something, then it's probably time to vary a workout slightly. The other thing that will influence a change in workouts is when you get bored. When you get to the point that your exercise programme is starting to become a bit tedious, you need to start thinking about switching pretty soon. A major benefit of cross-training, and of varying your activities throughout training cycles, is that this keeps you mentally fresh.

STRATEGY 4 PROGRAMME PLENTY OF VARIETY AND REST

Building in a mixture of different activities is a way of making the cycle of adaptation and progression work well for you. It's a way of creating a holistic set of physical benefits, and of letting your body recover between workouts so that you're getting the maximum benefit from each workout that you're doing. By allowing your body to recover, you can constantly be building on what you've done before, rather than driving yourself down into an exhausted state where you're not training at a level of quality. Training gets results, but quality training gets quality results.

Persevere

The hardest part of the whole game often lies in taking those first few faltering steps. Jackie points out that smoking research has shown the average person tries and fails six or seven times before they successfully quit. Building an exercise habit can be much the same.

---

* Part of the reason for this result is that lifting weights builds muscle and therefore the size of our fat-burning engine. Another factor may be that weight training utilises the a-lactic anaerobic energy system, a highly inefficient form of metabolism that creates a high-energy demand during the post-workout recovery period (more on this in Chapter 4).

Whether it's a team sport or running, swimming, tennis, yoga, dance or skiing, the first few times you do it might not be a very rewarding experience. But it *will* get better. Normally it will improve after just two or three sessions, as your body starts to recognise the particular set of movement patterns. If you can just hang in through those early days, you'll experience an incredible feeling when you begin to get some mastery of that sport. Success breeds success and you actually want to keep going because you feel you're doing well. Anyone who's had children will understand that when babies first learn to walk they fall over all the time. But no parent ever says, 'Oh well, walking doesn't seem to be your thing. Let's get you a wheelchair.' We encourage and praise our kids for every effort until they eventually find their feet. We have to extend that same gracious attitude to ourselves and give our bodies time to learn new skills.

The first couple of times I tried yoga ten years ago I hated it, really hated it. It was painful, it was too tough, it was boring — even BodyBalance, the modified version for regular people like me. Jackie wouldn't let me quit, of course, and by the third class I started to find it bearable — perhaps even grudgingly see some point to it. But around about my fifth or sixth class I underwent a magical transformation. I was hooked, as I am to this day. My weekly classes seem to make my body function as though it were 20 years younger, I enjoy the social interaction with the other regulars and I get a real aesthetic pleasure out of mastering the movements. If I had quit during those first few sessions I would have missed out on a whole new wonderful dimension to my life.

If you try something that you think you'd like to do but it's not as much fun as you expected the first time you do it, just take it easy and hang on in there. Always be as gentle on yourself as possible during those early sessions. Don't worry about what other people are doing. Persevere. The reward that comes when you start to get it is worth the extra effort and will spur you to keep going. It's a wonderful feeling when you start to feel the co-ordination, when you feel that you're mastering the challenge of a particular sport.

Keep setting challenges

Don't worry if you have a few false starts. If you try, and give up, a few times that's OK. Just pick yourself up, dust yourself off and start again. There are a lot of activities to choose from.

Our family loves to ski a lot now. You start off being able to do the green basic runs and then you work up to the blue runs and then up to the black runs and then you work up to being able to do the double black/yellow expert-only ones. And it's the same as everything else we've discussed in this chapter: there are feelings of achievement, that real reinforcement you get from setting a goal and then succeeding. Just being able to get down some of those runs is a big challenge.

When we ski in North America I love to compete on the Nastar courses, which are social races. It's a slalom course — you start at the gates, go round the flags and it's timed. You get to race against someone next to you and time yourself against thousands other people of your age. Given my complete mediocrity at the sport and with only around 20 days a year to change this reality, I understand that any goals I set are unlikely to amount to much. But taking part brings back the wonderful thrill of competition. The moment the start tone goes off, you are totally consumed: all the stresses of everyday life fall away and you become nothing but the race.

At first you're a hopeless learner, then you get to the point where you're able to ski, then you start working on your technique and gradually, over the years, you get to the point where you can get down some of the really difficult runs or enter a race. Every step of the way you get the incredible feeling that hey, I challenged myself and I succeeded.

There's huge positive reinforcement in this, a great feeling of independence and empowerment. That empowerment is a great thing — a personal sort of strengthening that you take into your everyday reality. You feel more capable of succeeding at work as well as with other goals — and life.

That's what's so wonderful about just competing in sports: you get all of that whether you really succeed or not.

The catharsis of competition

The first time you compete you'll probably experience terrible nervousness. Don't worry, that will disappear. Over time it will turn into exhilaration.

You'll probably experience plenty of failures along the way. Don't worry about those either. Experiencing failure is part of learning to succeed. Think of the babies learning to walk.

With tennis, when I played in my first small doubles tournament I was unbelievably nervous. It was strange: I'd competed for years on the track, often in front of big crowds; I'd gotten to the point where I just loved stepping out into the starting blocks. Here I was with about a dozen people in the stand and I could hardly hold the racket! I played appallingly and was soundly beaten. I was despondent after losing the match, but there's a strange and fortunate thing about competition . . . it somehow burrows inside you and gets you hooked. The next day the despondency was gone and I just wanted to do better next time. I realised the true difficulty of the challenge. I wasn't going to get any good by playing three days a week, so I started doing more. I entered some other tournaments and sometimes found myself training a couple of hours a day to get fit for them. Although I never got past being a B-grade player, every one was a personal growth experience.

Every time you compete, you see where you are; you realise what you've got to do to progress; you see where the next mountaintop is, the next peak. It's the time of truth and you understand where you've got to vary the mix. It becomes instantly clear what you need to do to actually achieve your next goal.

What's happening while you're doing that, of course, is that the competition is keeping you motivated and you're achieving peak physical health without even thinking about it.

STRATEGY 5 NEVER GIVE UP

Coax and cajole yourself through those difficult early stages. If you fail, don't worry; failing is part of learning to succeed. Keep trying; you'll get there in the end. It will be worth it!

Summary: just do it

Find a sport and set yourself a goal. That goal is what lifts you up and gives you incredible motivation to train, a reason for you to get out there and do it every day. Even if you're not planning on being the next Lance Armstrong, it doesn't matter; it will become part of you, and will ensure the sustainability of your exercise programme.

The goals will take you somewhere else: win or lose, you've changed. By the time you've competed in your first sporting event you're a different person. Even if you crash out badly, if you fail completely, it's not important. At that point you're a whole lot more knowledgeable, you've become much fitter and you're a motivated person. You're not the person who's failing every time they start to exercise; you're part of a system that is going to keep you involved in exercising for the rest of your life.

You'll experience an incredible sense of achievement and the joy of physical fitness. You will have solved the problem of being really out of shape and discovered a whole new way of being.❩

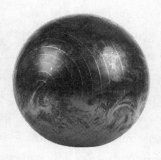

2 | **forever fitness**

Make your workout time your social time

jackie ❝ I never work out alone! Exercise is a fantastic way to keep in touch with people and to develop deep and wonderful relationships through shared experiences.

On Monday afternoons I meet with my sisters for a tennis lesson. They're both up to their eyeballs with kids and work, so this is the only chance I get to be with them regularly. We've permanently booked our long-time coach and friend Dave Knott for that time slot, so it's still a workout and a social outlet if one or more of us can't make it. Dave is constantly amazed at how much we can talk and still play; multitasking, we call it!

For years, on Tuesday and Friday mornings a group of friends have met for an early yoga session. Afterwards we go for coffee. I rarely get time to see these guys outside of this class and I love this chance to catch up; I always feel great for the rest of the day.

Thursday mornings I go for a two-hour power walk with my dear friend and colleague, Jenny Kruger. Jenny and I worked together for many years in obstetrics. She's currently doing her PhD in the subject so we talk about that and other aspects of medicine, plus all of the normal things women talk about. This is one of the absolute highlights of my week.

I'm fortunate to be creating and trialling fitness classes as part of my job, so I get to do all sorts of different exercise programmes during the company's quarterly cycle. But outside of those times I have regular sessions with PT Corey Baird and kickboxing instructor Doug Viney. Both of these guys are great fun and introduce a social break to my day.

If I ever feel that I'm getting out of touch with a friend, we schedule a 'walking meeting'. Phillip and I also walk together a couple of times a week and I believe that these times really enrich our relationship. And if we're having a 'discussion', no one can storm out!

Occasionally we get to go out with friends in the evening, but like most people these days we're very busy and what little spare time we have, we tend to preserve for family. So bit by bit we've designed our exercise time to become our social time. This has had the triple reward of ensuring that we stick to our exercise schedules, making our exercise more enjoyable and creating enough social time to stop us going insane (we hope).

phillip | On Friday afternoons, a group of my old friends and I get together at the Les Mills gym in Takapuna, on Auckland's North Shore. If the weather is good we'll jog down to Takapuna Beach and swim out to the buoy or do some gentle interval running on the beach. If the weather is bad we'll stay in the gym and do a weights workout or an indoor cycling class. Afterwards we grab the healthiest food we can find at the café next door and hang out for ten minutes before heading back to work. Like most people these days, we're all trying to do too much and are struggling to balance work and families, so we rarely get to see each other outside of this Friday afternoon session. It's one of the highlights of my week and I guard it jealously; don't even try to get an appointment with me at this time!

Mondays and Wednesdays at noon I meet my personal trainer and old friend Herb Chang at the Les Mills club in the city. Herb's been training me for around 15 years, so it's more like a social catch-up than a workout. Normally we lift weights, but if I don't feel like that we'll do a class or go for a jog and stretch in the park nearby. Once a month we have an appointment with our young friend Corey Baird, one of the new generation of super-qualified PTs. Corey does tests like postural assessments and gives us innovations to add to our workouts (about a quarter of which I actually do, but even so they really make a difference!). I love to chat with the other lunchtime regulars. Some of them have been coming in for decades and have also become like old mates.

On Saturday mornings I religiously attend a BodyBalance class in Takapuna. I always try to persuade Jackie or other friends to join me, but Saturday mornings have proved difficult for that. I've been doing the class for about five years and I've become acquainted with most of the other regular class members, so it's a real pleasure to catch up with them. This is the only time I see most of them, but they feel like old pals, and small groups of us sometimes get together afterwards for a coffee or a smoothie.

Sundays I play tennis or go for a run or bike ride with my one of my best mates, Peter Pearless. Our friendship goes back to track and field days — Pete was an Olympic 800 m runner for New Zealand — and it has extended into a business partnership. If the weather's bad we'll meet at the gym for a bike class, often with Jackie plus Pete's partner Sandy.

Last, but far from least, when we get a chance in the early mornings before work, Jackie and I go for walks or runs with the bizarre dog our daughter left behind when she moved out. We also regularly do classes together at the gym as part of our jobs. ❩

STRATEGY 6 MAKE WORKOUT TIME YOUR SOCIAL TIME

Call your friends and family members and plan regular workout times into your diaries. Book set activities like walking, visits to the gym, personal training and coaching sessions. (Personal training and coaching are much cheaper when shared between a few people.) This will dramatically enrich your life. Do it now.

Join a team

Modern society is increasingly isolating. We work long hours, often alone with our computer screens. We commute alone in our cars to work, and we live cocooned in our apartments or fenced-off properties. We commonly don't know our neighbours and even when we do, there's never enough time to talk or visit. As civilisation has become bigger and more urbanised, we've lost much of the family and community support we had just a few decades ago. This is very stressful for social animals like us.

In *You, The Owner's Manual*, Michael Roizen and Mehmet Oz make the radical statement that the mental and physical stresses of modern life artificially age the average person by 32 years. They present a list of remedies for this, based on the largest and most important scientific studies, and insist that the average person can win back around 30 of those years. At the top of their list is regular daily exercise, but not far behind are *friendship* and *social affiliation*. Loneliness is bad for your health. In the midst of our isolation, more and more people are craving community. There's been an upsurge in the popularity of social venues like gyms, new age churches, local cafés and online phenomena like *myspace.com*.

It's a primal thing, developed over the thousands of years during which we evolved into tribal creatures, banded together for protection against predators. We helped each other to gather food or hunt game, and shared in the pleasures of preparing and consuming the spoils of our labours.

There's nothing that satisfies these instincts like working out in a group and playing sport with a team. Working physically together for a common cause, sometimes against a common 'foe'. Sharing in the planning, the stalking and the gathering. Experiencing the joy of physical exertion, either at the steady rate of foraging or the accelerated rate of the chase, blood surging as the body works at its maximum, performing the functions for which it has evolved. We know this sounds like a purely male thing, but it's not. While historically men did more hunting than women, this wasn't universally the case. There have been many female hunters and warriors throughout history, and the genes aren't all that different. Modern women are a great example of this; try taking on Mia Hamm on the soccer field, guys, or Maria Sharapova on the tennis court.

Whether it's a social soccer or touch football league, a serious training group preparing for a triathlon, or just a walking/jogging group of friends who compete in the occasional 10 km fun run, there's a wonderful bond that forms when you train with a team, and the camaraderie adds a huge dimension to the exercise experience.

We've lived in many different cities and countries around the world and wherever we've gone, we've found that the quickest way to make real friends is to join a local tennis club, running group or fitness class. When you're working out with people, sharing powerful physical experiences and endorphin highs, you tend to open up, to be a lot more authentic with each other. There are no politics, few hierarchies, and bonds tend to form more quickly than they do at work. Bonds formed with teammates are lasting and powerful, not unlike those formed between squad members who fight alongside each other in battle.

Choose the right team

While we say there are few hierarchies in sport, respect in the eyes of your peers is still important, so consider this when you're deciding which sport to pick up and which team to join. As adults, we tend to do things that we were good at as kids; we tend to find sports and careers that we've had some success at, and where we've had some social reinforcement. Knowing that you are a valued member of the tribe, or team, is a critical part of wanting to stay with that group, so when you're choosing a sport try to pick one that you have some aptitude for, maybe something you did when you were younger. The basic neural patterning for most sports is developed between the ages of 9 and 13. This means your brain has been programmed for that activity, so you'll have a head start if you choose it again when you're an adult.

Alternatively, pick an activity you've always wanted to try, but find a social team or beginners group and build up gradually. You don't have to be the best, just reach a comfortable level where you can keep up and feel good about what you're doing. As your expertise grows over time, your enjoyment will be increased by the small signs of admiration and acceptance you get from the other members of your team.

You can find teams to join at your local sports club, university or gym. Sports equipment or sportswear shops can often recommend them and city councils or community organisations usually have good local lists. As with anything these days, you can frequently find what you're looking for online.

> jackie ❛ It's great to put together your own team — of friends or workmates — and enter a local social league or inter-company competition. A few years ago my sister, Janine Phillips, organized a group of 17 people from the firm of stockbrokers where she worked and entered several teams into a corporate triathlon. Some of them had never played any serious sport in their lives. Over the four months that they were preparing for the event, a fantastic team spirit grew and this carried over into their workplace. They became an incredibly motivated team who loved working with each other, which dramatically improved their commercial results. The company's management was thrilled and made it an ongoing part of their business operation. ❜

Getting over the initial fear

A lot of people are too insecure to join a team. They fret that they won't fit in or won't be good enough. Don't be worried. Feel the fear and do it anyway, because once you get in there you'll find lots of people just like you. We've seen this literally thousands of times over the years. Some gyms have a reputation of being only for the super-fit, but people are constantly amazed that when they finally get up the courage to step over the threshold, they find a wide range of body types and levels of fitness.

If you're joining a gym on your own, one of the hot trends these days is Small Group Training. You'll find everything from specialised sports training to weight loss groups. They'll be run at set times —normally for six weeks — with six to twelve people in each group and dedicated professional coaches. These small group sessions are a great way to fit in and make friends.

STRATEGY ⁄ JOIN A TEAM

You're never alone. There are all sorts of people who share your aspirations and almost everyone's got the same insecurities. If you take the plunge and persevere until you

get over the hump, you'll find it is incredibly worthwhile. Nothing will enhance your enjoyment of exercise as much as this. Nothing will help you stick to your exercise programme as effectively. There are few things you can do that will enrich and extend your life as much as becoming part of a sports or fitness training group.

Get a personal trainer or a coach

If you're feeling shy about starting a sport or joining a gym, it's always easier to get a friend to go along with you. Gym research shows that people who join with family or friends attend more regularly and stay on as members for much longer. If you just can't make that happen for some reason, then think about hiring someone. PTs can really smooth your induction into the gym. They'll get you confident with the exercises, write you an expert programme that's tailored specifically to your body and your needs, and they'll help create a schedule you'll stick to. Best of all, a trainer will be a friend who helps you through the intimidation most people feel when they enter a new social environment. Likewise, a tennis coach or a surf or ski instructor will help you to create a sustainable routine for those sports.

Personal trainers

Over the next few pages, we offer you some inside tips for using personal trainers, based on our experience in the fitness industry and as passionate users ourselves. Fifteen years ago, there were virtually no PTs in the world; a few celebrities had them and that was it. Now there are hundreds of thousands and they are a commonplace part of modern life. This is a remarkable cultural phenomenon.

As John Naisbitt predicted in *Megatrends* in 1982, as people become wealthier they are starting to put more value on non-material things like their health. If you're earning $50,000+ a year, why shouldn't you spend a few thousand protecting your most precious asset? Even if you earn less than that, you can afford a few sessions to get you started properly.

In the old days, when you joined the gym a lowly paid and often underqualified gym instructor would give you a basic weight-training programme, a quick session on how to use the equipment and leave you to it. Clubs simply couldn't afford to do any more than that. Members paid an annual fee of a few hundred dollars, and it was financially impossible for the average gym to employ sufficient instructors to give constant coaching and care to everyone. In the past 15 years, personal trainers have stepped in to fill that gap and have solved a huge problem for the fitness industry.

phillip (We nervously introduced the first personal trainer in our Auckland city club in 1992. Wendy Smith (now Sweet) was a highly qualified operator, skilled in cardiac rehabilitation for wealthy businessmen who could afford her services. All the same, we feared screams of protest from our members at the prospect of being asked to pay for programming and fitness advice that had previously been free. We were amazed to find that she was immediately inundated, not with rehab work but with regular people wanting fitness and weight loss programmes. We added another trainer, then four more and within two years we had 20! Now there are 90 full-time PTs working out of that gym alone and demand is still growing.)

These days, a well-qualified trainer with 20 to 30 clients can earn from $50,000 to $100,000 a year. Clients pay anything from $50 to $5000 annually, depending on the frequency of their workouts (sessions typically cost around $30 for half an hour and $50–60 for an hour). Compare that to the old-style gym instructor, who might earn from $20,000 to $30,000 per annum.

These income levels, together with the positive lifestyle, have attracted highly qualified, experienced people into the profession. There are coaches from a huge range of sports, physical education teachers, practitioners of alternative therapies like yoga and Pilates, and now a whole new wave of people coming out of the specialist training courses set up at polytechs and universities to service the demand. In some clubs you'll even find former doctors who have decided they can get more satisfaction from helping clients to improve their health than writing prescriptions for sick people. A good personal trainer can make as much money as the average New Zealand GP and they tell us it's a much more enjoyable environment in which to work.

With the wide variety of training programmes and different types of trainers available, you have a huge range to choose from. Many gyms get every new member started with two or three sessions with a trainer, or they'll offer a discounted introductory package. We strongly recommend that you take these up: they're well worth the investment of your time and money. A trainer will help you set your goals — the long-term ones that give you the ongoing motivation we talked about in the previous chapter — then they'll write an exercise programme for you. If you continue past the introductory period, they will work with you day by day to achieve maximum results.

But it also becomes a social thing. Personal trainers usually become friendly with their clients. Your trainer will help you through the initial period in the gym when you're a newcomer and you're feeling a bit alienated. If your budget is tight you can just catch up every few weeks or months to get your programme updated. But if you employ a trainer on a regular basis you'll get to know each other well and your training sessions will start to become a great social experience as well.

Choosing the right trainer

Making friends with your trainer is great, but you're still paying them to help you get results. If you want a fast fix to get in shape for a big event like a wedding or your sports season, you'll want a trainer who'll push you hard. But in the long term, we believe it's important to train at a level that you enjoy. You might sometimes feel like being pushed, but at other times you'll be exhausted from work and life and you'll just need a maintenance dose.

If you find your trainer regularly pushes you harder than you would like, then talk to him or her. Explain that you need this to be sustainable for you, and you don't want to work out like that. Likewise, if you're bored, make it clear that you want to enjoy the sessions and you'd like more variety. Feel free: you're paying for the service. If you think that somebody is just not right for you, that's okay too. There are a lot of great trainers out there — try different ones until you find somebody you click with.

When you're choosing your trainer, first decide what you need, then try to identify a PT who fulfills the requirements. Some are motivators and educators; others are good counsellors; some of them really know how to have fun with their clients. Different trainers also have different areas of expertise. Most prescribe a combination of weight training and cardio work as fundamental components of any programme for fitness and weight loss (we talk more about the details of this in Chapter 4). With weights, some just programme the traditional exercises for muscle building or fat loss, but others are qualified in advanced exercise for functional improvement — you might have heard labels like core training and stability training. Pilates and some types of yoga can also be used for this. At the cardiovascular fitness end, most will prescribe walking, jogging, cycling, stair climbing — or their equivalents on the machines in the gym — plus a variety of fitness classes. Others specialise in a range of outdoor activities, stretching from team sports to triathlons or canoeing (some are *experts* in certain sports). There are also a number who are specialists in nutrition and diet.

Trainers normally have one area that is their passion, plus one or two 'bread and butter' secondary qualifications. Most gyms can give you profiles on their different personal trainers. You can talk to the fitness director or the personal training manager and they will help you to identify the PT who is going to be just right for you.

The benefits of a good trainer

An expert trainer will take you through the various forms of exercise in your programme repeatedly, teaching you the correct techniques until you have mastered them. They will not only maximise the results you get from the exercises, but minimise your chance of injury. Unfortunately, injuries are a part of any sport or exercise programme. But the vast majority of these are minor and short term — infinitely preferable to dying of a heart attack or other obesity-related illness. Learning expert technique will minimise sports injuries *and* reduce your chances of suffering from chronic pain brought on by non-sport causes such as osteoarthritis at any stage of your life.

If you do have pain, some highly qualified trainers specialise in cutting-edge rehabilitation techniques that are becoming an increasingly preferred alternative to surgery. Look for people with qualifications like Paul Chek diplomas or advanced Pilates certification — these guys can dramatically improve your life.

A good PT will put together a workout programme that involves activities you enjoy and builds your fitness at a level you can handle. This encourages long-term exercise adherence because you're much more likely to stick to a routine that you enjoy. Your trainer will typically change your programme regularly to avoid plateaus. Once your body adjusts to the exercise in your programme it learns to work more efficiently and this means your results level out. Some trainers tell clients that you have to 'shock to unblock' — so a good trainer will always create a mix of activities that will give you the benefits of cross-training and keep your body guessing about what's coming next. Each session, your trainer will check how you're feeling and try to gauge the level of intensity you're up for. They'll ask standard questions about what you had to eat for breakfast, how well you slept, that kind of thing. A trainer's not a mind-reader though; you've got to provide the information. Again, if you ever feel that you've been pushed to the point of not enjoying your training, then say so.

You can have a personal trainer anywhere. If you're seriously overweight and you're embarrassed to go to the gym you can get someone to come to your home and get you started. Better still, get a group of friends together and hire one: it spreads the cost and makes the workouts more fun. During Phillip's Friday afternoon sessions at Takapuna Beach he often sees personal trainers coaching small groups of women, who look as though they're just beginning an exercise programme. They do gentle intervals up and down the stairs and jog or walk on the beach, just exercising outdoors in the sun. It's a good start.

People often ask us what the most important reason is for using a personal trainer. The real answer is the appointment in your diary: it makes you show up for a workout. Never underestimate the importance of this simple factor. If you can afford to use a trainer on an ongoing basis, even a couple of times a week, this will keep you exercising regularly when all else fails.

Coaches

The gym is by no means the only place to get expert advice: the same principles apply to any sport. When Phillip started playing tennis in the early 1990s, we had a tennis coach coming around to the house, initially just one day a week; that became two, then three days a week. He had a succession of coaches until he hired Bruce Derlin, who was the national Davis Cup coach. At a different level, Jackie and her sisters meet weekly with their tennis coach for a social workout.

When we decided to take up surfing again as born-again teenagers, we hired a surf coach to get us past the embarrassing beginner stage, and we regularly use ski instructors. It's the same with any sport. If you're training for swimming, you'll be able to hire a swim coach at the pool. You'll be able to hire a cycle coach through your local bike shop. Go online to find someone in your area for your chosen sport.

Professional sportspeople all use them. Nowadays, most even have a technical coach *and* a trainer for conditioning. But coaches and trainers need more than one or two professional clients to make a living, and you can often hire these same experts no matter what your ability.

Any time that you've got an appointment with a coach that you have to honour, and he or she is teaching you technique, motivating you and providing some social interaction, you're doing something really good for yourself.

STRATEGY 8 GET YOURSELF A TRAINER OR COACH

Whether it's just for a few sessions to get you started, or as a lifelong companion — a trainer or coach is a great investment in sustainable exercise. A great one will change your life. Get a few friends to join in and it's cheaper and even more fun. Start shopping now.

● | **INSIDE THE MIND OF A GREAT PT**

A trainer we know, Jacinda (Jac) Faloon (now Cavendar), was renowned for her ability to really understand the needs of her clients and the importance of linking exercise into their existing lifestyles. She had a client, let's call him Mr Smith, who trained with her at 6 am three times a week. He was a busy corporate executive with grown-up children and a wife he adored.

Regular exercise was new to him and he soon found that

the sessions at the gym were doing him the world of good, but — and it was a big but — he no longer had the energy to join Mrs Smith for their regular Friday afternoon round of golf. Some trainers might have told him not to worry; his gym sessions were getting him much better results (and besides, they wanted the income from three sessions per week). When he shared his predicament with Jac, her response was immediate: 'You'll have to stop seeing me on Friday mornings. I won't let anything come between you and your golf with Mrs Smith.' She understood the importance of his family support and his role in encouraging his wife with her exercise activities.

A few months later Mr Smith's son was getting married and wanted to improve his fitness before the big day. Who do you think he chose as a trainer? You bet. Jacinda. And when Mr Smith's daughter-in-law-to-be found out that her fiancé was spending his time in the gym with a lovely young trainer, do you think she was concerned? No, because she had heard how much Jacinda respected the bond between Mr and Mrs Smith. In fact, she started exercising with Jac too, working on losing some extra kilos before her wedding.

Throughout this whole time, Jac had never met Mrs Smith. That year, Jac held a Christmas picnic for her clients and invited them to bring along their families and friends. Here's how she describes that event:

'It was a stunning Auckland day and I hosted the picnic at the magnificent property of friends of mine. There was a long, sweeping driveway and right on time at 1 pm I saw a beautiful late-model car slowly pull up the drive. I was a little

> When he shared his predicament with Jac, her response was immediate: 'You'll have to stop seeing me on Friday mornings . . .'

intimidated because I knew it was Mr and Mrs Smith and I was nervous about meeting her. I knew her husband so well and had worked with her children, but I really didn't know how she felt about Mr Smith getting out of bed so early twice a week to work out with me at the club.

'You won't believe what happened. The car door opened and out stepped an immaculately groomed women wearing a gorgeous suit and a lovely summer hat. She walked confidently towards me and as I prepared to shake hands with her, she reached out her arms and enveloped me in a tight embrace. As she pulled away she looked me straight in the eye and said: "It's wonderful to meet you, Jac. Thank you for everything you have done for my family." That was one of the nicest moments of my career. I have always believed that families who play together, stay together and that affirmation gave me deep satisfaction.'

Support your partners

The more social support systems you can build around your exercise regime, the more chance you'll have of making it a part of your lifestyle and therefore a lifelong habit. But social support networks are two-way streets.

At a simple level, if you want your life partner to live long and healthy, and to be pleasing to your eye, then you need to support him or her in their pursuit of that. We love the Dr Phil story about how his wife, Robin McGraw, hands him his tennis bag when he gets home from a trip and tells him not to come back until he's done some exercise. She supports his desire to get out and play tennis regularly and encourages him to maintain his routine even when he's been busy and they haven't had enough time together. She knows it will make him healthier, less stressed, and a better husband and father.

Make a pact with your partner, family and friends that you will support each other in your exercise regimes.

Team motivation

At a more sophisticated level, let's consider team motivation.

Research has been conducted among US soldiers fighting in the Middle

East into what makes them put their lives on the line in battle. It turns out that while they often cite factors like national ideals, the main reason they fight is for each other: that is, to support the members of their squad. Sports teams are much the same. Powerful bonds are formed and members will make great sacrifices for their team mates. Witness the brawling at top professional level when a member of the opposition attacks a player on a football team.

The more you can build that team spirit, the more powerful the support will be for everyone's individual success within the team. Some of the things you can do to help create this are:

- Be there. Demonstrate your loyalty to the team by not missing sessions. The more commitment you show to the team, the more powerfully they will support you. If they don't, then look for new team members who will.

- State your personal goals and honestly share your motivations for having them. Whether you dream of achieving a certain time or ranking in your chosen sport, or you just want to get into shape, don't be afraid to share it with your team mates.

- Motivate your team mates by reminding them of their goals and congratulating them when they reach a milestone.

- Find a coach you all respect and want to perform well for.

If you can, create a higher ideal. It's always a great motivation for your team to be training for a charity race that will involve people donating money to a good cause, based on your mileage or some other measurement of performance. Or try just stating a mutual philosophy, like supporting each other in helping to create a sustainable future by minimising the strain on our health system.

STRATEGY 9 SUPPORT YOUR FAMILY, FRIENDS AND TEAM MATES IN ACHIEVING THEIR FITNESS GOALS

Lead the way; start changing the world in your back yard. The more you give, the more you'll get and the better shape your world will be in.

● | **IN THE LES MILLS ORGANISATION, OUR GROUP FITNESS TEACHERS HAVE A CREED THAT GOES AS FOLLOWS:**

We are the warriors in the battle against sedentary lifestyle

We are here for the people in our classes

We honour our programme, our peers and our club

We keep ourselves in peak physical condition

We love music and exercise

We welcome feedback

We create magic fitness experiences

We strive to be star performers and remain team players

By inspiring positive change in our classes we can change the world

We both really believe in this. It is a moral purpose that drives us to give our maximum for this company, and research among our more than 60,000 teachers shows that they love being part of this mission.

Healthier, happier and less materialistic

We've covered making your workout time your social time, joining or creating a team, hiring personal trainers and coaches, and becoming a support hub: all great ways in which you can help create sustainable exercise regimes for yourself and your friends, family and colleagues — *and* enrich your lives in the process.

There's the healthy stress-release and fun you have working out with friends, the social reinforcement you get from holding up your end and doing things well in the eyes of your peers, the strong social bonds that form with team mates and the deep communication that occurs when you share physical and emotional experiences with people.

We believe that people whose deep emotional needs are fulfilled through exercising together experience a lesser need to replace that fulfillment with overconsumption and material acquisition.

The more you can make fitness a social thing, the more likely it is to become something you do long term, and the better the quality of your life will be.

For many people, visiting the gym after work is becoming what going to the pub or a bar was for earlier generations. Exercise will give you highs through the release of endorphins and other biochemical delights. It's the same sort of buzz that you get from downing a drink or two — but it will be a hell of a lot better for you in the long term.

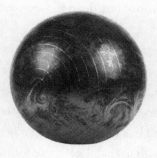

3 | **it's a game of inches**

In our experience, people start an exercise programme half a dozen or so times in their lives before they succeed in making a habit of it. So far we've discussed two powerful ways to beat those odds: setting big hairy audacious goals that inspire you to change your life (and working up to them through a series of small, practical steps), and transforming your workouts into enjoyable, social experiences with friends, team mates and coaches.

In this chapter we're going to talk about a third big strategy, which is to minimise the pain and effort by doing everything we can to make exercise *fun*. We'll go through a range of activities and hope you find one that's right for you. But first we'd like to give special and particular attention to one very important activity that can have a huge effect on our environment: cycling.

On your bike!

Ditch the car! One of the very best things you can do for our planet, your health and the level of absolute joy in your life is to start walking or riding a bike to work.

In developed countries, around 20 per cent of emissions of carbon dioxide, the primary culprit in global warming, come from cars. (This does not include commercial trucking, which accounts for another 13 per cent.) In 1996, according to a study on gridlock by Texas A&M University, it was found that drivers in Los Angeles and New York City wasted 2270 million litres of gas annually while just sitting in traffic, going nowhere. That translated into about 6.8 million tonnes of carbon dioxide in those two cities alone!

phillip ' I ride my bike to work two or three days per week. Any time that I know I don't have to travel from my office to meetings in other parts of town, I cycle to work. It's only about 20 minutes each way, but cycling has significantly increased my fitness and lowered my body-fat percentage. I take a slightly longer route with less traffic, but I often get to the office more quickly than when I drive. More than that, I get there feeling fantastic.

When I drive, I often arrive at work feeling stressed and angry from battling the traffic. And when I go home, it gets worse. I'm already burnt out from a long day at the office and the rush hour traffic becomes nearly intolerable.

When I cycle, I get home feeling energised and empowered. I have a relaxed glow and am completely recovered from any stress that's accumulated at work. On the bike I feel really alive: in touch with my environment, in contact with the elements, my body moving physically with a strong, natural purpose. I'm relieved not to be trapped in a car.

If you decide to take up cycling, it's important for safety and comfort that you have the right equipment; choosing it can be a lot of fun. There's all sorts of new technology around bikes and cycling apparel. I have a road bike with carbon fibre bits here and there to lower weight and vibration and improve feel, plus tyres with a tough Kevlar component to minimise puncturing. My bike has slightly upright handlebars instead of the normal racing ones that have you uncomfortably hunched over.

I know serious racers who are really passionate about the whole subject of their equipment. Anyone with friends who cycle will know exactly what I mean.

Your local bike shop can advise you on this stuff and is a great place to get information about cycle groups, races and coaches.

You'll need a backpack to replace your briefcase and to carry some extra work clothes. This can be difficult with formal clothes. Although companies are becoming more relaxed about staff wearing casual or active wear to work, the best thing a business can do to encourage employee fitness is to install a locker room, or at least some showers. I keep a pair of shoes and a few spare clothes at the office, which I replace on the days that I have to take the car. **)**

Mountain biking

jackie **(** We also keep cheap mountain bikes at various work locations around the world. One of the workout highlights of our lives is cycling around the forest trails near Aix en Provence in the south of France. Aix is the home of our good friend Christophe Andanson, an ex-Olympic wrestler who dropped 10 kg, became an aerobics teacher and is now our company's exclusive distributor in France. It has been our European work base and we have lived there from time to time since 1997.

Around Aix you can ride past ancient vineyards and fields, through the forest to a 2000-year-old Roman watchtower, or along a ridge facing beautiful Mount Saint Victoire, once home to the painter Paul Cézanne. You can smell the lavender of Provence, watch the jet trails disappearing into clear blue skies over the Luberon and the Vaucluse, and imagine the Gauls, Romans and Moors who once travelled these roads. In the summer it's usually too hot to ride during the day so we ride in the early evening and often encounter deer and wild boar along the trails.

Mountain biking anywhere, and everywhere, is a buzz. The exhilaration of difficult terrain or the liberating feeling of just being able to go wherever you want is addictive. And there are places all over the world like this. If you look around you're sure to find one in or near your town, even in big cities. Our company has an office in Aliso Viejo in Orange County, southern California. Phillip was working there for three months in 2005 and we did some biking around the beautiful surrounding hills. Even just riding along the estuary at Newport Beach was nice. In New Zealand, my sister Janine and I occasionally drive out to Woodhill Forest near Auckland, which is a wonderful playground for thousands of mountain bikers. **)**

Cycling is superb for your heart and your waistline and there are so many fun ways to do it. Another really enjoyable version that has become popular is bike classes at the gym.

Bike classes

Serious cyclists have conducted indoor cycling classes using road bikes on rollers for decades. But South African Johnny G popularized the modern class, introducing Spinning™ to the world in the early 90s using a special stationary bike. It created a revolution in gyms.

phillip When I started on the gym floor in the 1970s, we had funny little stationary bikes with a speedometer. It was one of the most boring exercise activities ever invented. We used to put magazines out for people to read while they pedalled, but it was still difficult to get anyone to stay on long enough or pedal hard enough to do themselves much good.

In 1981 we imported some sleekly designed space age contraptions from Germany called Dynavit cycles that incorporated computer technology, giving users simulated terrain variations like hill climbing, along with digital feedback. Popular versions of these, such as the Lifecycle, soon flooded the world's gyms. These bikes were much better than the old speedometer versions, but realistically it was still a pretty boring way to work out.

The late 80s saw the arrival of the Cardio Theatre. You could sit on your bike in front of a bank of TVs screening different channels, tuning your earphones to whichever one you wanted to watch. This was a big step forward in terms of fun and got a lot more people exercising. It also made it easier to cycle for longer. But when Spinning arrived it blew everything else out of the water.

The concept and equipment are simple: a stationary bike, heavy for stability, with a resistance knob that you dial up and down, standing for 'hill climbs' and sitting for 'sprints'. What makes it so good is that you have a teacher urging you on, great music suited to the rhythm of the ride, hip studio décor, and an intimate group of people around you, simulating a *peloton* or pack ride. You end up burning two or three times the number of calories you would by yourself, and it's fun. You get to know people in your class and can organise weekend road rides if you're interested.

I have a commercial interest in cycling classes; our company has its own branded bike class, RPM, which is taught in about 3500 gyms around the world. But of all the classes we produce, this is one of my favourites and I take part in it regularly outside of work.**)**

Cycle tours

When we're visiting a city briefly on business, we look for bike or walking tours, which are a great way to experience a place and maintain a little bit of fitness while you're travelling. Bus tours are unbearably boring by comparison.

Guided bike tours are also becoming more popular. You cycle through the countryside from venue to venue and the tour company brings your bags along behind. Another variation is to cycle from vineyard to vineyard. It's a fabulous way to exercise and see the world. A friend of ours sold his business in his early 40s, and every year for the past decade he and his partner have spent months riding around the countryside in Europe.

Safety

For all the great benefits of cycling we have to recognise it has some real and serious dangers. Be sure you have a good-quality, very well-fitting helmet and good gloves to protect your hands. You can also get specialist safety gear for mountain biking, such as wrist- and shin-guards. The main thing is to pay strict attention at all times. While there is the odd idiot on the road, most drivers are very courteous to cyclists. The cycling accidents we have had have been through our own inattention.

Later in the book we'll discuss our recommendations for what governments should do to encourage cycling and make it safer for people. Let's hope that in the very near future we'll see some action on this score. In the meantime, be careful out there.

If you can't ride, walk

We'll talk later in this chapter about walking and hiking as separate activities, but most of the things we've said about cycling apply to walking. Commuting on foot is a wonderful way to begin and end your work day and makes an excellent contribution to the health of the planet.

STRATEGY 10 RIDE A BIKE

Do the environment, your health and your sanity a huge favor by walking or riding a bike to work, on at least a few days a week. Cycling is a great fun activity that's fantastic for your heart and your waistline. You can get involved with racing, as discussed in Chapter 1, or a club or training group as discussed in Chapter 2, and you can find a way to enjoy it at any age.

Find a favourite sport

If you want to make exercise fun, then the logical place to start is by choosing activities you enjoy. Let's start with sports. As we said earlier, if there is one that you liked as a child then see if you can find an adult league. Or try something new. Think of what you enjoy watching on TV, or what you've always imagined yourself playing. Otherwise, think of something you can do with your children or with your friends. Just dream for a moment.

Sports used to be largely the domain of the aristocracy — the original purpose of amateurism was to keep the working classes out. Now it's available for *everyone* in an increasingly wide range of choices. As you've gathered by now, we and our friends are completely sports-mad — we try anything and everything! Here are ten great options for you to consider, beginning with a few we've already talked about, then moving on to some wilder options:

1. Team sports

If you enjoy watching football on the box — rugby, soccer or gridiron — and you'd like to take it a bit further than just vegetating on your sofa, there are plenty of options available. Look on the web for local touch football leagues or visit your local soccer club. These days there are social and mixed leagues everywhere. Touch football has gained incredible popularity around the world over the last 20 years — ten per cent of adult New Zealanders currently play it. Once regarded as a junk sport, it now has national and international tournaments. Whether you want to play in serious competition or just have fun, it's excellent for your fitness.

Basketball is another great option. Join a team or just front up at your local pickup game at the gym or the park. Women's basketball and netball have also grown tremendously in recent years; statistics show that ten per cent of adult New Zealand women play netball.

Hockey and volleyball are other great team-fitness sports and many cities, even those that are landlocked, run beach volleyball leagues in summer. As we discussed in Chapter 2, the greatest thing about team sports is the team!

jackie | I played netball (outdoor basketball) throughout my school years. My sisters and I went back to it in our 30s, playing in a social league, and loved it. My older sister Sue still plays in a mixed team with her husband and other family members.

Phillip played rugby league through his teens and tried social rugby when we lived in Sydney. Injury knocked him out pretty quickly, though; I think touch football is a better option for adults.

2. Running

If you see yourself as the next Hicham el Guerrouj or Paula Radcliffe, you can take your first faltering steps by entering a local fun run and preparing for it the way we described in Chapter 1. Your local track club, gym or sports-shoe store will help you find a coach and a training group. If it's sprinting or field events you fancy, the number of people involved in masters-level athletics is now many times larger than regular track and field. There are track meets every year, all around the world, where thousands of over-30s gather for competition — and socialising!

phillip | My old college roommate, Los Angeles attorney Jason Meisler, was a 7 ft 2 in [2.18 m] high jumper in 1976. Thirty years, one open-heart surgery and two knee operations later he's still going. I made the mistake of racing him and my son, Les, up the track stadium steps at UCLA last year and they both killed me. Les is a fast, fit junior basketball player and the amazing thing is that Jay beat *both* of us! After the heart scare he changed his life and now keeps himself in peak shape by working out at the track every day.

Orienteering, mountain running and cross-country are all great variations on this theme. There are many fun and semi-serious races around the world every year, from your local 10 km fun run to the New York Marathon.

3. Tennis

If you get a buzz watching Roger Federer or the Williams sisters, go and join your local tennis club and take your first steps on the road to the top.

> phillip | I once played against a 47-year-old in the Fiji Tennis Open who was the World Masters Champion for the 45–50 age group. He owned a retail business in Melbourne and had worked hard his entire career. Then he decided that he was going to add some spice to his life and took up tennis. He became very committed and trained every day for a number of years. He didn't have a particularly brilliant technique, but he trained very hard and became a world champion. (Needless to say, he wiped me off the court.)
>
> Tennis has a real Zen to it. Every time you reach a new level, you see the next couple of levels above. You don't understand what a tactical game it is until you achieve a basic proficiency and start to make your shots with reasonable consistency.
>
> Whenever I played doubles with my old coach Bruce Derlin, once ranked 67th in the world as a doubles player, he would say stuff like: "You stand here . . . three shots from now you're going to take a forehand volley." The complexity of the tactics and court geometry involved in tennis make the game physically and mentally addictive.

4. Hiking

You'll get healthy, have some great social interaction and it's a treat for the soul. Organise your family or friends, choose a variety of interesting routes or venues and just do it. Simply walking around the streets near your home or in a nice park is a great way to stay fit. But there are some more serious options.

Our company has a lot of overseas guests who visit in groups. We often take them hiking through the Waitakere Ranges, out to ruggedly beautiful North Piha beach on Auckland's west coast. The Waitakeres are a subtropical rainforest just 30 minutes' drive from downtown, with some areas of prehistoric vegetation. We sometimes come across hiking club members out for day-long treks. Their members are always friendly and they take regular weekend hikes in all sorts of beautiful locations.

jackie ❛ For a student holiday job I was once an assistant guide on the Routeburn Track in the South Island. Hiking is something I've been passionate about all my adult life and am starting to do more of. Janine and I recently walked the Queen Charlotte Walkway in the Marlborough Sounds. It was a stunning four days filled with great exercise, conversation and scenery. We also hike in the Waitakere Ranges in Auckland.

I strongly recommend this as a pursuit to take up at any stage of life. The bush, birds and other wildlife are so good for our souls. One year we took our children and their friends on the famous Milford Track. They all came out with a huge appreciation of how beautiful New Zealand is. This has got to be good for city kids!

Our local bookstore owner, Andrew Maben of Novel in Herne Bay, goes trekking every year in places like the Himalayas. He trains seriously to get into shape for these adventures and has had some incredible experiences. It's a great way to see the world.

For your entrée to wonderful outdoor experiences, you'll find lots of local hiking clubs listed on the web; for trips further afield you can also talk to your travel agent.

An interesting and humorous book on the subject is Bill Bryson's *Walk in the Woods*, his account of walking North America's Appalachian Trail — a hike that from beginning to end can take months! ❜

5. Golf

Play golf, but never set foot in a golf cart. This means being able to afford a caddy — or being prepared to lug your clubs around the course yourself, which is an excellent thing to do. Most people can play just as good a game with half a dozen clubs in a light pack.

Golf has all the right elements. You're out with your friends in beautiful surroundings. It's a great long-way-around sort of exercise. Just don't go near that cart: it's a killer.

6. Swimming

Most local pools have an adult swim squad that trains before work or in the evenings. Adult swim competitions have become very popular and many cities also have mass harbour swims. It really is a thrill.

Just training is a great source of enjoyment. It can be tough when you start, but once you begin to develop your technique it's a beautiful, rhythmic feeling. Being in the water at the local pool has a magical aesthetic all of its own and it's easy to get hooked.

There are all sorts of water sports that you can get involved with, like water polo, or even offbeat things like underwater hockey.

phillip | I played water polo for a couple of years and it's one of the most enjoyable sports I've ever tried, combining the fun of being in the water with the excitement of rugby. And it's fantastic for your fitness.

7. Skiing

Skiing is one of the real adrenaline-producing sports, and you don't need to get competitive if you don't want to. The pure pleasure of gliding down a mountain is a sort of spiritual high. Equally, you can get *really* competitive about it and that makes more of a lifestyle commitment.

As we discussed in Chapter 1, there are all sorts of social or adult competitive skiing options. Bill Robertson, one of the founders of our global business is a former top-level swimmer and has been one of the Australian national swim coaches. His son Matt is a professional downhill skier and Bill takes several months of the year off work to support him around the world. Bill skis in adult competitions himself at the same time and describes this as one of the best things he has ever done in his life.

Most of us don't have lives in which skiing all year round is possible, but when you combine it with summer sports it's a great seasonal option.

jackie | My good friend Janet Alexander lives with her British husband Chris in San Diego. We went through Phys Ed school together. After being inactive and in the corporate world for years, Janet changed her life and has become one of the world's leading personal trainers. Chris is a triathlete and Janet, being fabulously competitive, joined him in this. Within a few years she was winning events in her age group, and they went on to compete in the winter sport of biathlon, whch is a combination of cross-country skiing and shooting. She is now a world-renowned athlete in her 40s, still in top shape and "not looking a day over 30".

8. Triathlon

Triathlon and other multi-disciplinary events have been among the most inspired sports inventions of the last few decades. From the first triathlon in San Diego in 1974 (short course) and Hawaii in 1978 (long course or Ironman), the event has grown to be a great Olympic sport, with hundreds of thousands of competitors of all ages worldwide.

Our Auckland gym introduced triathlon to New Zealand, holding the country's first event in 1979. We organised national championships and other events until the mid-80s, when a national association was formed to take over the growing workload. It was a big investment of time and energy for us, but incredible bonds were formed among hundreds of people, most of whom are still members of our clubs. We, and most of our friends, trained together for triathlons and it was a wonderful time in our lives.

There's a wide range of events all over the world now, from standard triathlons to all manner of multi-sport events and adventure races like the world-famous Coast to Coast (243 km) in New Zealand's South Island. Thousands of people take part, from top-level international athletes to school kids starting out or office workers just wanting to enjoy the sport.

Its cross-training aspect makes triathlon one of the ultimate fitness sports. Many triathlons are run just for women and these have proved incredibly popular for first-timers. Your local gym, swim club or bike shop are good places to get started.

jackie | My dad was still competing well into his 60s and just loving the social environment of the training and of competition day. My brother-in-law Paul Bowskill is the same. A corporate executive by day, his triathlon hobby has led to him competing in the Hawaii Ironman three times!

9. Diving

Every summer for 15 years as our children grew up, we and a group of friends rented two beach cottages on the eastern coast of Great Barrier Island — home of some of New Zealand's most beautiful beaches. We'd spend every day hiking, bodysurfing and diving. We love snorkelling and would sometimes cover miles of coast. As you get more and more into it, you start to go for hours and it becomes excellent exercise. You can gather shellfish or crayfish and feed the family at the same time!

Anywhere we go that's got a beach and warm water, we find a reef or a rocky coast and go out with a snorkel to look around. We've also scuba dived for years. You can get started at a holiday resort, when it's often more convenient to do a course than at home. Being underwater is like being on another planet. It's a fantastic get-away-from-it-all stress release and if you work hard at it, it helps keep the holiday kilos off.

10. Board sports

jackie ‘ I *love* windsurfing and Phillip likes sailing Hobie cats. It's great exercise and a huge thrill. Again, its something you can get started with on vacation, or head down to your local sailing club.

Surfing is another sport that our family has got into on holidays. Phillip surfed as a teenager but I never did. The kids and I started by going to surf school at Waikiki. We got hooked on it and now it's become another regular healthy holiday activity.

Many adults are getting back into surfing and that's a good thing. It's fantastic for your fitness and once you get started it's a real addiction. It's also a wonderful way to exercise when you're on holiday and going for a run seems like too much of an effort. ’

And much more

There are dozens of other sports options that might suit you:

- In addition to tennis you can try badminton, squash or racquetball.

- Rollerblading and ice-skating are fun and great exercise.

- Martial arts are excellent for your body and your self-confidence. White-collar boxing is becoming increasingly popular. You train for three months to go into the ring in front of a crowd of friends and supporters. It's just three, two-minute rounds, with full head-guards and oversized gloves (the right safety equipment is very important — don't participate without it). Boxing is very intense and builds up a high level of fitness, plus self-confidence and an enormous sense of achievement.

- Rowing, kayaking and canoeing are fantastic fitness sports which are currently undergoing a new surge of popularity.

- Indoor and outdoor climbing are two of many other excellent options.

Open up your imagination — there's a sport out there for you. And just about all of them have organised clubs where you can give it a go before you invest hundreds of dollars in the gear.

phillip — Some years ago a bunch of friends and I had a paintball team. You run around in the forest for a few hours every weekend trying to capture other teams' flags. The secret to success at the game is to move fast and non-stop. It's exciting and exhausting, and when you make a mistake and take a paintball in the chest it's fun . . . in a primitive kind of way.

Looking back over the past few pages, I realise some of this may appear frivolous and egocentric. But for us, over the years, this has represented a serious battle to stay healthy. As you age, you have to keep coming up with new ways to make being active fun.

STRATEGY 11 FIND A FAVOURITE SPORT

Finding something you really enjoy doing is a good way to create an exercise habit and sports are great for that. As we said in strategy #1, once people get hooked into a sport they forget about having to motivate themselves and actually start to look forward to their next session. They get excited about the chance it provides to improve, to move closer to their goals. The exercise becomes secondary to the passion of taking part, improving and learning new skills.

Find a great gym

We have an obvious commercial interest here as gym owners, but our years of experience in the field give us insights that we hope you will find helpful.

For a huge number of people these days, the gym will be part of their fitness solution — either as a means to supplement their sport or as the place where they do most of their exercise. As society becomes busier, it's a convenient, time-efficient place to exercise. And gyms are the best place for weights workouts, a key part of training for health, weight loss and almost every sport.

In 2006 in the United States, 41.3 million people had health club memberships. Add to that the approximately 20 million Americans who use corporate, university or hospital-based facilities, or just attend a club casually, and you have over 20 per cent of the population going to the gym (at least periodically). That is more people than are playing golf, tennis or any other sport. The gym is becoming the biggest exercise venue in the Western world.

Gym membership in the US has doubled within the past 12 years. However, the number of gyms there has doubled within the past *six*. Most developed countries have seen similar trends. Our city of Auckland, with a population of more than 1.3 million, has seen an increase from around a dozen clubs in 1980 to over 150 now!

The growth in supply has created intense competition in the industry over the past few decades, resulting in a dramatic improvement in products and services. Clubs are constantly looking for an edge over their competitors. When one introduces an innovation, others jump on board quickly, with the exercise equipment industry striving to fuel this fire.

'Exertainment'

The description earlier in this chapter of the evolution of exercise bikes is a good example. Gyms have moved from the old wind-resistance speedometer model to computerised bikes, Cardio Theatre and then Spinning classes. In addition to bikes, clubs have introduced a phenomenal range of stair-climbers, treadmills, elliptical walkers, rowers and cross-country ski machines, with all sorts of graphics from bio-feedback to virtual reality, and new innovations every year.

In 2000, we started opening 'cardio cinemas' in our clubs in New Zealand. These rooms are like movie theatres with a big screen, surround sound, non-stop music videos and 40–50 cardio machines.

Health club architecture is evolving rapidly, with a strong move towards 'experiential' design. In the 1990s, the Crunch chain from New York started to build gyms with outrageous décor and nightclub lighting. Since then hip urban gyms have opened around the world, like the L'Usine in Paris, The Third Space in London and David Barton, whose New York and Chicago clubs are like chic ultra-lounge bars.

The Amsterdam branch of the UK's David Lloyd chain has a whole gym done up like a Las Vegas sports bar, with four enormous movie screens showing sports and music videos. Our Les Mills Auckland City branch has a half-million dollar theatre stage, lighting and sound system in its main group fitness studio, which hosts classes of up to 200 people in a dance party atmosphere.

The market is spreading in all sorts of directions, from small, niche, women-only clubs like Curves to huge category-killers like Lifetime Fitness in the US and Virgin Active in Europe. Some clubs have moved towards high-end luxury and others to peaceful, natural looks.

There are plenty of choices, from big and buzzing to small and intimate. Find a club with an environment you enjoy — somewhere that makes you want to work out and which makes you feel as though you belong there.

Personal service

There's also been a revolution in gym services. The personal training explosion described in Chapter 2 is a classic example; in place of the old gym instructor scenario, you can get as much one-on-one help as you're prepared to pay for, from a rainbow variety of different experts.

Another example is club communications, which have been transformed by the electronic age. One by one, clubs around the world are picking up on new technology and using it to build education and community among their members. Our friends Lynne and Victor Brick have a chain of clubs called Brick Bodies based in Baltimore. Their members receive an email stream of inspirational health tips and motivational notes with headings like 'Message From Good Ole Uncle Vic', designed to keep them on task with their fitness.

More and more clubs have web forums where members can make suggestions, ask questions or just talk to each other. This and other trends like small group training are helping gyms get better at providing the friendship that people have traditionally found in sports.

In the end, service is all about people and culture. The ideal club is one whose staff are genuinely passionate about helping people get healthy and fit. Shop around. A club with the right people can change your life.

Group fitness

Easily the biggest force in making gyms more fun has been the group fitness revolution. As we mentioned, when Spinning classes came along they revolutionised the exercycle.

It's the same with other gym activities. What started in the 80s with aerobics has evolved into a whole new generation of classes, as the industry finds ways to make exercise more and more entertaining. Everything from weight training to martial arts to alternative mind/body activities like yoga, Pilates and t'ai chi. There are step classes, army-style boot camp classes, and dance classes from ballet to hip hop. They've all been put to music and converted into a modern way of moving.

Tae Bo, the class by Billy Blanks that made kickboxing famous in the late 90s, is an example. It transformed a traditionally disciplined niche activity into one that's now enjoyed by millions of people; they get not only great fitness but confidence and empowerment.

Lifting weights has evolved into BodyPump, which we created in our living room in 1990 and has become the biggest branded fitness class in the world. The principle is the same: powerful instructors, loud energising music and a party environment have replaced the discipline required to pump iron by yourself in the gym. You perform hundreds of repetitions of all the basic barbell exercises, hardly noticing the pain.

According to the Australian Bureau of Statistics, participation in fitness classes grew by over 300 per cent between 1996 and 2001. In the United States, fitness classes are the fastest growing sector of the gym industry.

To get started, select an activity that appeals to you. There's a huge variety to choose from; you've got all the athletic options, but you've also got gentler, low-impact versions for older people and beginners.

Take it very easy the first few times — *don't* try to keep up with the regulars. If you start with BodyPump, use just the bar for the first few sessions, or maybe add some very light weights. If you select a cardio class, cruise your way through your first few sessions, or set a goal of lasting for three songs and then build up to five and so on until you can aim to make it right through to the end. It can take a few weeks to get used to the exercises if they're new for you, and to the sheer volume of work — even if you're reasonably fit. If you make it easy on yourself and hang in there for a few classes it'll start to feel great and then it'll get addictive, which is what you want.

STRATEGY 12 FIND A GREAT GYM

To maintain good health, you need to work out almost every day. Unless you're involved with a group of friends in a sport that involves you doing this, then you're going to have to find supplementary tricks that keep you motivated. A good gym will do this in many different ways — and will help make your training fun.

● | **A CENTURY OF FITNESS**

The fitness boom started at the end of the 19th century, in response to increasingly sedentary lifestyles brought about by the industrial revolution. By the 1920s, 'physical culture' clubs were booming, featuring activities such as weight lifting, calisthenics classes for men and women, and the now-forgotten 'Indian clubs' (large iron clubs like bowling pins that were swung in various configurations to improve physique and endurance). Early strongmen and bodybuilders like Eugene Sandow and Joe Greenstein were well-known in their day. In America, Bernarr McFadden published the first physical culture magazine from the turn of the century through to the 30s, inspiring early fitness revolutionaries such as Bob Hoffman and Don Bragg, who

> The fitness boom started at the end of the 19th century, in response to increasingly sedentary lifestyles.

some of our parents and grandparents will remember. Phillip's great uncle, Norman Kerr, operated one of New Zealand's first physical culture clubs, the Glengarry Institute, in the 1920s and 30s.

The movement died during the Great Depression and World War Two but started to make a comeback in the 50s and 60s, inspired by people like bodybuilder Charles Atlas, fitness guru Jack Lalanne and magazine publisher Joe Weider.

Then, all of a sudden, whether as a result of health-related publicity or just fashion trends dictating briefer clothing, the general public started getting fitness-conscious.

In the 70s we had the jogging boom and our club ran jazz dance and calisthenics classes. But in 1980, when we started modern aerobics classes, people went crazy.

To begin with, the classes were held in a little studio that could take a maximum of 30 people. Within weeks we had to move to a room that would hold 40, and then to one that would hold 80. Within a year we bought the building next door to allow us to convert our main gym into a 150-person studio. Finally we were forced to build a room on the roof that would hold 300 people.

We built gyms and held classes all over New Zealand, and then Australia; everywhere we opened we'd have crowds of people. There was a queue around the block when we opened in Christchurch. We remember launching classes in Dubbo, an Australian country town, and 600 people turning up at the local town hall.

Originally it was mostly women in leotards, but we found that there seemed to be no limit to how athletic we could make it. BodyAttack, a tough cardio workout that we created in 1980 under the name JazzErgetics, is now taught in clubs all over the world. Throughout the 80s we introduced dumbbell classes and circuit classes with weight training equipment, and finally in 1990 we introduced BodyPump, which is now attended by millions of people worldwide.

Over the past few years we've been involved in organising increasing numbers of 'fitness parties', a new global phenomenon. As many as 10,000 people pay to attend a day of back-to-back classes featuring 'rock-star' instructors, with full-on rock-concert sound, stage and lighting systems.

Lean and strong, a whole new breed is developing out there — people who would look like aliens from another planet to Great-Uncle Norman's generation. This is one of those rare modern trends that feels good!

Other tricks for making it fun

Start where you feel comfortable

An important part of making exercise fun is to ensure it's not embarrassing or hard: start where you feel comfortable. There's nothing more off-putting, for example, then trying skiing for the first time with gun skiers who insist 'You'll be fine!' on the harder runs and then swoosh off ahead of you. It's embarrassing and it's hard, and you may never go back.

phillip (I shared this part of the book with a friend of ours who has a lot of experience in getting people started in exercise. She just about blew a gasket. "Unbelievable," she said. "You have just described my first time skiing and it was *you*, Phillip, who sped off down the slopes of Coronet Peak in Queenstown, leaving me stranded with no way down. It was late in the afternoon and the chairlifts had all stopped so I couldn't even thumb a lift down that way. Eventually, a ski patrol came across me firmly planted on my butt in one of those 'not even a forklift could move me' moods, and cajoled me down the mountain, one awkward wedge turn after another." Our friend is now a handy snowboarder — her determination to master snow is a reminder that you should never give up. Apologies, Sach!)

Wherever you start, you have to do it very gradually. You have to avoid doing anything that's going to give you an aversion to fitness. You have to make it fun or you won't go.

Take the jogging example. Don't start by trying to break the four-minute mile by running around the block as fast as you possibly can. You'll come back exhausted and in pain and for the next few days you'll hurt like hell. You've got to start at a level that you enjoy. Start by walking. As we've said earlier, get a group of people together, or go with a member of your family or a friend. Spread the word around and put regular times in your diaries to ensure that you're going to do it. Resolve to support each other.

Pick a scenic route. Walk along a beach or through a leafy park. Do it on a nice day, in the sunshine. Maybe plan to finish up in an area with a lot of cafés and give yourself the treat of a nice (low fat!) coffee once you've finished your walk. Then build from there.

Choose something you feel comfortable with, but don't be afraid to begin. When you do, you'll be surprised at how many people are in the same situation as you. Even the real fitness-fanatic gyms are very different on the inside. People are always surprised when they venture in: you get a huge variety of shapes and sizes.

You'd be surprised by how many people say they don't want to join a gym because they feel too overweight, which defeats the purpose, really. You have to move past this.

Everyone's been a beginner at some stage, everyone remembers how hard it is, and people actually respect you for getting started. People have a funny self-consciousness: they think they'll be ridiculed. Personally, when we see an older, overweight person out walking or jogging or in the gym, we have nothing but admiration for them. We just think, 'good on you for making the effort'. And we hope that people extend us the same courtesy when we try new activities.

Mix it up

Cross-training is another key. We discussed plateaus in Chapter 1 — how your body adapts and you need to keep challenging it. But this has a psychological dimension as well: you need constant variation within your workout programme so you don't get bored. Set yourself a work schedule that has different times, different distances, different speeds and different intensity levels. If you're at the gym, lift weights one day and do a yoga class the next. Choose different terrains and different landscapes if you're running or biking. Really mix it up and make it fun.

Ideally, you should mix and match your activities so they complement each other; keep a good balance between strength-based activities and cardio work. There are good ways that you can mix activities between the gym and sports, and there are also a lot of activities that you can train for at the gym but enjoy outside when you have the time. It's common for people to do cycling classes in the gym during the week when they're short of time, and over the weekend go out for a good long bike ride in the countryside. A change of scene keeps it fun and doesn't let your busy schedule rob you of your exercise.

Buy an iPod

They're good-looking as well as being the must-have technology of the moment; now you have a real excuse to get one. In a study conducted at Fairleigh Dickinson University in New Jersey, researchers found that adherence to a weight-loss walking programme was significantly greater when the participants wore headsets and listened to music as they walked. We prefer social forms of fitness but if you must do it on your own, get wired for sound.

Listen to talking books

jackie **❢** One of my dearest friends, while recovering from surgery for breast cancer, knew she had to exercise to keep herself sane and increase her chances of optimal recovery. So she started walking. To get through the initial pain and boredom of it, she rented out talking books from her local library to listen to as she exercised. This not only got her through her walks, but became a life-changing experience.**❞**

Start competing

There's nothing like the anticipation at the start of a race. You're competing against the person next to you and you can feel their nerves. You're waiting for the clock to tick down and the gates to open. You're standing alone with your ability and your body.

Competing is fabulous for personal development — the reinforcement that you get from beating challenges and reaching little goals along the way. Whether you fail or succeed, there's a self-affirmation that goes on psychologically.

It's incredibly exhilarating and it's also fun — and addictive. The longing for that rush is the best motivation to get out there and train. It's an experience of being all that you can be — of being totally alive. And when you finish, you'll have achieved something that no one can ever take away from you.

Capture the joy

There's a whole aesthetic dimension to physical activity that we've barely touched on. With each sport there's a different wonderful feeling when you master it. Feelings of having everything working as it should be . . . of strength, of grace, of being in perfect control of your body. You won't get it right all the time but the overwhelming sense of satisfaction you get from doing something well, even once or twice, is enough to keep you coming back for more.

Most recreational golfers make lots of mistakes but the bliss that comes from hitting a drive down the middle of the fairway sustains them through the next five holes of abject misery. And when you finally catch a wave and ride it all the way to the beach, you'll be hooked on surfing for life. Discovering the essence of movement in sport and exercise activities can be like a spiritual experience — and for some people it is.

Whether it's tennis, dance, yoga or just moving beautifully on your morning run, learn the techniques from someone who knows, perfect the form, and you'll unleash the transcendent joy of movement that takes you right out of the frantic pace of everyday life.

STRATEGY 13 MAKE IT FUN

The more fun you make your exercise regime, the longer you'll keep it up, and the fitter and healthier you'll be. As Phillip's father, Les, says: 'You have to find a way to fall in love with fitness.' Find your path, aim to live as long as you can, and enjoy it to the max!

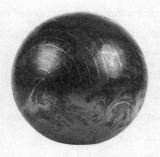

4 | free the mind, the body will follow

Expand your knowledge

This may seem like a strange way to begin a chapter about exercise, but we have to confess to a long-term love affair with wine. What started this was a book by Robert Parker that a friend gave us for Christmas one year.

You begin reading those wonderful descriptions of different wines from around the world and you want to try them. You taste a few, you read a bit more, then bit by bit you start to develop some knowledge around the subject and it becomes a hobby — a part of your lifestyle*. Knowledge has its own way of breeding motivation.

---

* In case you're thinking that reading this gives you an excuse to become a drunk, hard luck, that's not the case. Most research says that a glass of wine a day is good for you — or even two for men. However it also states that if you drink more, there are health risks instead of benefits. We normally limit ourselves to one or two glasses a night, two or three nights a week.

Fortunately, this principle doesn't only apply to indulgences. It's the same with any hobby, including sport and exercise. The greater your expertise, the more confidence and motivation you'll have, the better your results will be and the more you'll enjoy it — and therefore be likely to stick with it.

Exercise involves reading!

If you're just getting started, we recommend that you get hold of a good book on your chosen sport or fitness pursuit. You'll feel a lot more expert, which will help you get over any initial self-consciousness. You'll achieve better results because your energies will be correctly focused. You'll pick up some good pointers on technique, which will increase your enjoyment and lower your chance of injury. And perhaps best of all, you'll have an ongoing source of motivation to fall back on when you hit the rough spots that are common when you start out.

As part of your long-term programme, we recommend that you read all you can.

It's simple these days to go to an online bookstore and find the most popular or highly recommended texts. Amazon or Barnes and Noble have good ratings and reviews.

The publisher Human Kinetics specialises in sports and fitness. Most sports also have journals you can subscribe to. These provide a constant source of motivation and renewal of interest. The internet is packed with sites that offer inspiration, education and online forums where you can discuss challenges and share successes with others who are at your level.

In the general fitness field, we love books like *Younger Next Year* by Chris Crowley and Henry S. Lodge; *You, The Owner's Manual* by Michael Roizen and Mehmet Oz; and Miriam Nelson and Sarah Wernick's *Strong Women* series. They're written in an enjoyable, motivational style that makes us want to get out and exercise more.

The more you learn about something, the more that knowledge enriches your whole experience of doing it, and the greater your motivation, confidence and enjoyment.

Get coaching

Get as much coaching as you can, especially during the crucial beginning phases. Good coaches help minimise the period when you feel like a stupid learner! It doesn't have to cost much: as we noted in Chapter 2, tennis or golf coaches, ski instructors and even personal trainers all provide much less expensive group lessons as well as individual tuition. Experienced friends are great too: ask them for advice.

The other big benefit of coaching is that it helps you develop great technique.

Great technique equals great results

The better your technique, the further you can go; the better you can be with the sport and the more enjoyment you can get out of it. As mentioned in Chapter 1, Tom Tellez, arguably the world's greatest track and field coach, was a stickler for technique.

phillip ❜ Tom preached perfection. He would explain the optimal bio-mechanics of a movement. When you're running, for instance, your arms should swing forwards rather than across your body; if they swing too much across your body, you are directing force sideways instead of straight ahead. For optimum speed you want all your energy being directed straight ahead down the track.

He coached using images, which are the most powerful way to teach any sport. That's because, putting it simply, the part of our brains responsible for co-ordination works in pictures rather than words. Tom would talk about elbows bent at right angles, arms swinging like a pendulum from the shoulder. I remember him picking athletes up for something as small as a hand flapping during their arm swing, which would cause some minute amount of energy wastage.

Anyone who remembers seeing Carl Lewis run will know what I mean. Tom's athletes were poetry in motion and their results reflected that. ❜

Good technique helps you avoid injury

Good technique also helps you to avoid injury, and serious injury is one of the things that can curtail your involvement in a sport. With any sport, if you want to be able to do it long term, great technique is an excellent base.

Some injuries are simply accidents, caused by a tackle or a fall. But many are over-use injuries, which come from repeating a simple movement thousands of times, incorrectly. As we age we become more and more susceptible to this, because our production of things like immune cells and tissue-regenerating hormones starts to slow down in our early 40s, making us slower to heal.

Our good friend, Auckland orthopaedic surgeon Garry Heynen, is one of the world's leading hip specialists, one of the developers of mini-incision hip replacement. He considers that much joint deterioration among active people is due to poor technique, often resulting from muscular imbalances around joints.

Garry points out that no movement is produced by a single muscle — there are at least seven muscles, for instance, involved in knee flexion and extension. He believes that people starting a new exercise programme or sporting activity over the age of 40 should begin by strengthening their muscles to balance joints. For this he recommends exercises like weight training, Pilates and yoga, emphasising the importance of strengthening opposing muscle groups.

An example of this might be, rather than just doing pushing exercises to develop our pecs, we also need to do pulling exercises that develop our upper back muscles and balance our shoulder joints. Or rather than just working on our abs, we should include back exercises. Try to build in leg flexion as well as leg extension, etc.

There are simple protective things you can do with technique for most sports. For example:

- If you're running or walking, imagine there are headlights on your hips — you want to keep them perfectly aligned forward, on full beam. This is a powerful image that will tend to keep your legs tracking correctly, protecting you from knee and ankle injury.

- For aerobics, dance, weight lifting, walking, jogging, yoga and many other upright activities, imagine you're a puppet with a string coming out of your head that's pulling you upright. Keep your chest lifted, a *slight* curve in your lower back and your lower abdominals sucked in (think from time to time about sucking your pelvic floor inward and upward.) This posture will align your body correctly and protect you from many injuries.

You can learn the techniques specific to your sport from a book, a coaching DVD or, better still, a real live teacher or coach. Tennis elbow, for instance, can be avoided with simple racquet grip adjustments that can be shown to you by a good club pro. Many racquet sport players also tend to move incorrectly around the court, risking hip injury by lunging at the last minute for balls instead of moving early into the right position. As well, there's a tendency to run around the court stiff-legged, especially when we get tired. Instead of absorbing shock naturally in our knees and ankles, we start to absorb it in our hips.

Even one match played with poor technique can cause hip soreness. Repeated thousands of times, this can lead to hip deterioration and eventually the need for a joint replacement. It's essential that tennis, squash and racquetball players learn good technique — body square on to the net, knees bent, weight on the balls of the feet — and a good pro will teach us drills that make sure this becomes ingrained. This is called unconscious competence — it just happens without you having to think about it.

There are essential techniques for all sports, which we need to learn if we want to participate in them on a lifelong basis.

In addition to good basic technique, players of vigorous competitive sports are turning more and more to stability or core training, which we'll talk about later in this chapter. They're finding that this gives them greater protection — even from accidents and contact injuries — *and* improves their performance.

STRATEGY 14 EXPAND YOUR KNOWLEDGE

Read everything you can get your hands on about your chosen activities and get as much expert help as you can from professional coaches or experienced friends. This will create motivation and results, and will enable you to keep exercising all your life.

We've devoted the rest of the chapter to increasing your fitness knowledge in areas that we believe will motivate you to work out, beginning with . . .

Twenty-three reasons to exercise

There are thousands of studies out there that show the benefits of exercising. Lack of exercise, of course, is the main cause of obesity. But here are a few other reasons, some of them lesser known, that should help get you off the couch.

1. Exercise staves off dementia

Exercise will reduce the possibility of developing dementia and Alzheimer's. In 2004, the *Journal of the American Medical Association* (*JAMA*) reported that the strongest factor in maintaining cognitive function as people get older was undoubtedly exercise.

In February 2006, the *Annals of Internal Medicine* reported that those who exercise the most are at least risk of developing Alzheimer's. The study reviewed all scientific data on age-related cognitive loss in 20,000 women over the age of 20 and found that exercise was the most protective factor in maintaining brain function.

In January 2006, the online edition of *Neurobiology of Ageing* revealed that research conducted at the University of Illinois with 54 post-menopausal women demonstrated that brain atrophy was not an inevitable consequence of ageing. There are several ways — like exercise, a good diet and staying mentally active — that can slow or stop the process. Dr Kirk Anderson, the author of the study, wrote that the women in the study who scored higher in cardiovascular fitness maintained greater brain tissue volume and better test scores than women who were less physically active.

Another issue of the *Annals of Internal Medicine* (17 January 2006) reported that a research survey involving 740 men and women aged 65 or older found that exercising three or more times a week can reduce the risk of dementia and Alzheimer's by up to 40 per cent.

The question here, of course, is just how this works. In Madrid, researchers at the Cajal Institute believe they've discovered how exercise fends off the risk of Alzheimer's and other diseases of the brain. In the December 2005 issue of *The Journal of Neuroscience*, they reported that regular exercise can double the production of megalin, a brain protein that ejects a potentially destructive protein called amyloid beta. Amyloid deposits are well known in Alzheimer's patients: they accumulate in clumps throughout the brain.

2. Exercise makes older people stronger

There is a lot of research showing that declines in exercise efficiency and capacity of adults over 60 are reversible. The *Journal of the American College of Cardiology* (March 2006) reported on a study showing as much as a 30 per cent improvement in exercise efficiency and capacity after six months of regular exercise.

In a University of South Florida study, a group of people with an average age of 83.5 did 16 weeks of exercise; they made significant improvements in strength, mobility, balance and agility. How cool is that? It's never too late to get started.

3. Exercise prevents breast cancer

In a 12-year study of 90,000 women in France, reported in the *Journal of Cancer, Epidemiology, Biomarkers and Prevention* (January 2006), researchers found a 38 per cent lower risk of breast cancer among women who reported five or more hours per week of vigorous physical activity.

What is particularly fascinating is that the threat is lower regardless of other risk factors like weight, family history, the use of hormone replacement therapy (HRT), or a woman's reproductive history. It didn't matter if women had a family history of breast cancer. This same study showed 'a linear decrease in the risk of breast cancer with increasing amounts of moderate and vigorous exercise activity'.

4. Exercise makes you live longer

The pioneering Framingham heart study of 5206 people over a 46-year period found that of those who reached age 50, the group who engaged in high physical activity lived an average 4.2 years longer than the low physical activity group. The moderate group lived 2.3 years longer.

We're not talking here just about length of life: the same study showed that the high physical activity group had a better *quality* of life as well.

Another 2006 report in *JAMA* stated that people maintaining four simple health habits have a 69 per cent lower death rate from cancer and a 73 per cent lower death rate from heart disease. The most important habit was regular exercise. The other three factors were: not smoking; maintaining a Mediterranean-style diet with lots of fruit, vegetables, unprocessed grains, olive oil and fish; and taking a small nip of alcohol on most days.

5. Exercise helps your heart, whether you're fat or thin

This one's obvious, but the statistics are still scary and thinner people don't necessarily get off scot-free. In a special issue of the American Heart Association's *Circulation* magazine in January 2007, researchers noted that the incidence of heart disease among trim women who do not exercise is 150 per cent higher than it is in slender women who exercise regularly. There's a sliding scale, essentially, with trim women who exercise regularly at the top and those who are overweight and don't exercise at the bottom. Among obese women who do not exercise the incidence of heart disease is 340 per cent greater than it is among lean, active women. For women who smoke, are obese and do not exercise, the incidence of heart disease is 940 per cent greater than it is for lean, active, non-smoking women!

6. Exercise reduces abdominal fat — and fat is toxic

Another 2006 article in *JAMA* reported on research conducted at Northwestern University, involving 17,500 patients over 30 years. It found that being overweight in mid life substantially increased the risk of dying of heart disease later in life. The article said: '. . . fat tissue is a dynamic organ that is continually producing hormones and chemical messengers that increase the risk of blood clots and cause insulin resistance.'

In October 2005, the *Journal of Applied Physiology* revealed that a study conducted at Duke University Medical Centre had shown that just three hours of brisk walking a week could prevent the accumulation of deep abdominal fat. The build-up of abdominal fat was linked to a higher risk of type 2 diabetes, high cholesterol and heart disease. Exercise now, said the lead researcher, Dr Cris Slentz, and you might not be 20 pounds heavier in five years.

7. Exercise heals

Regular exercise speeds the healing of wounds in older adults by up to 20 per cent, which reduces the risk of infection. An Ohio State University study — recorded in the *Journal of Gerontology* in 2007 — reported that among people aged between 55 and 77, the body's ability to heal wounds is faster in those who exercise than in those who don't. On average, complete healing occurred in 29 days for the exercisers against 39 days for the non-exercisers. This is important: the faster a wound heals, the less it is exposed, and the less chance there is that it will become infected.

8. Exercise improves your sex life

Good news all round. Daily exercise is strongly associated with better erectile function in men. *JAMA* reported in 2006 that male health professionals between 51 and 87 who exercise vigorously for half an hour a day are half as likely to suffer from erectile dysfunction as men with the lowest activity levels.

And for women? The November 2005 issue of the *Journal of Sex Research* reported on a study conducted at Penn State University which found that the more a woman sees herself as unattractive, the more likely she is to report a decline in sexual desire. These results support a link between body image and sexual response. The women with negative body images 'especially dislike their stomachs or abdomens, hips, thighs and legs'.

A month earlier, research presented at the North American Association for the Study of Obesity showed that women involved in a weight-loss programme experienced significant increases in both sexual desire and in feelings of being sexually attractive. After only moderate weight loss the percentage of women in the study who felt sexually unattractive fell from 68 per cent to 26 per cent. The percentage of women who experienced problems with sexual desire fell from 54 per cent to 39 per cent.

9. Exercise can prevent and even cure type 2 diabetes

A report in the November 2005 *Journal of the American Association of Occupational Health Nurses* noted one university study in which the majority of diabetic and pre-diabetic patients in a two-year diet and exercise programme were no longer diabetic.

Young women who exercise in the year before they become pregnant greatly reduce their chance of developing gestational type 2 diabetes. *Epidemiology* reported in January 2006 that a study at the University of Washington found that women who exercised vigorously during that time frame reduced their chances by 81 per cent; women who exercised moderately reduced their risk by 59 per cent.

10. Exercise helps your joints

There's clear evidence that exercise is the best way to look after your joints, and can help repair them if you wind up with problems.

According to the Harvard Medical School's weekly health newsletter, there are six ways to prevent knee and hip problems like bursitis, tendonitis and osteoarthritis, and to treat them while they are mild. The first way is to stay active. The newsletter says: 'The knee was designed to bear weight, but it wasn't designed to go it alone. Strong flexible leg muscles take a great deal of pressure off this joint.' And there's more: 'Exercising your knee causes synovial tissue in the joint to produce synovial fluid, which lubricates the knee and nourishes cartilage.'

In February 2007, the website *www.webmd.com* noted that regular exercise confers many benefits on arthritis patients. One: it helps maintain normal joint movement; two: it increases muscle flexibility and muscle strength; three: it helps people to maintain a healthy weight, and in doing so reduces pressure on joints; four: it helps keep bone and cartilage tissue strong and healthy; and five: it improves endurance and cardiovascular fitness.

Basically, it said, 'a range of motion exercises progressively stretch the joints further until normal or near normal range is achieved and maintained. In addition to preserving joint function, exercise creates strong muscles, which helps keep weak joints stable and comfortable and protects them against further damage.'

Finally, exercise can maintain and even increase bone density. Researchers at the University of Arizona conducted a study which concluded that women involved in a routine of weight bearing and resistance exercises did not lose bone density over time — in fact they *increased* it by one to two per cent a year.

All of this means that you can help your body fight arthritis and enjoy a better quality of life as you age. In December 2005, *Arthritis and Rheumatism*

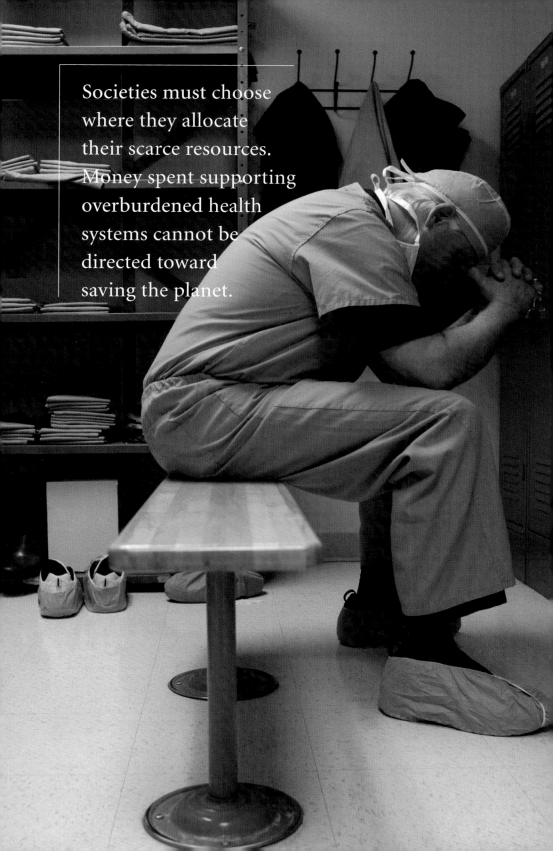

Societies must choose where they allocate their scarce resources. Money spent supporting overburdened health systems cannot be directed toward saving the planet.

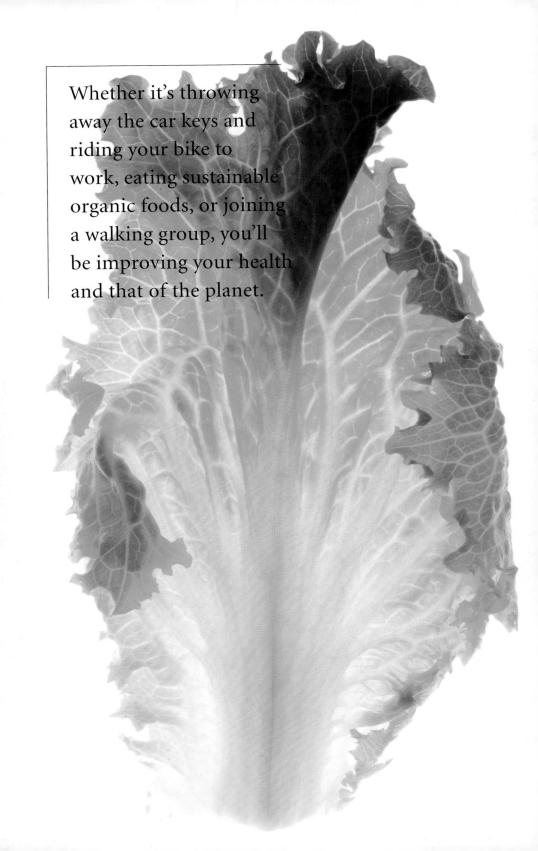

Whether it's throwing away the car keys and riding your bike to work, eating sustainable organic foods, or joining a walking group, you'll be improving your health and that of the planet.

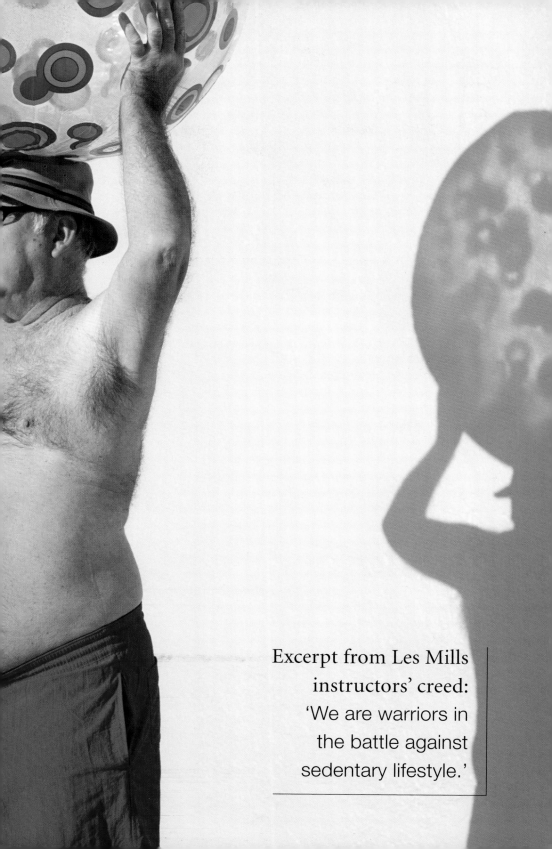

Excerpt from Les Mills
instructors' creed:
'We are warriors in
the battle against
sedentary lifestyle.'

People whose deep emotional needs are fulfilled through exercising together experience a lesser need to replace that fulfillment with over consumption and material acquisition.

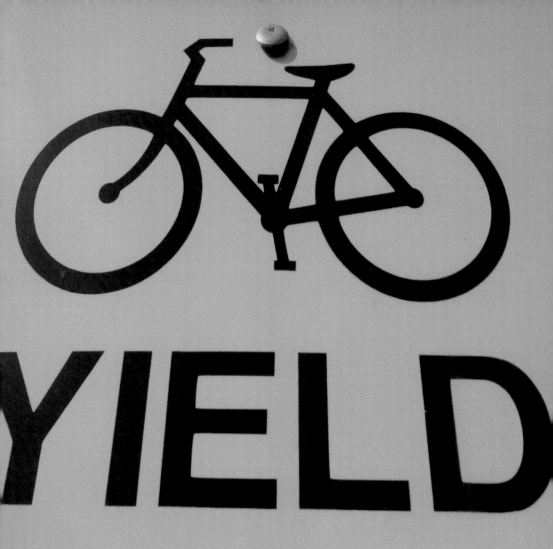

YIELD TO

One of the very best things for your health and the level of absolute joy in your life is to start walking or riding a bike to work.

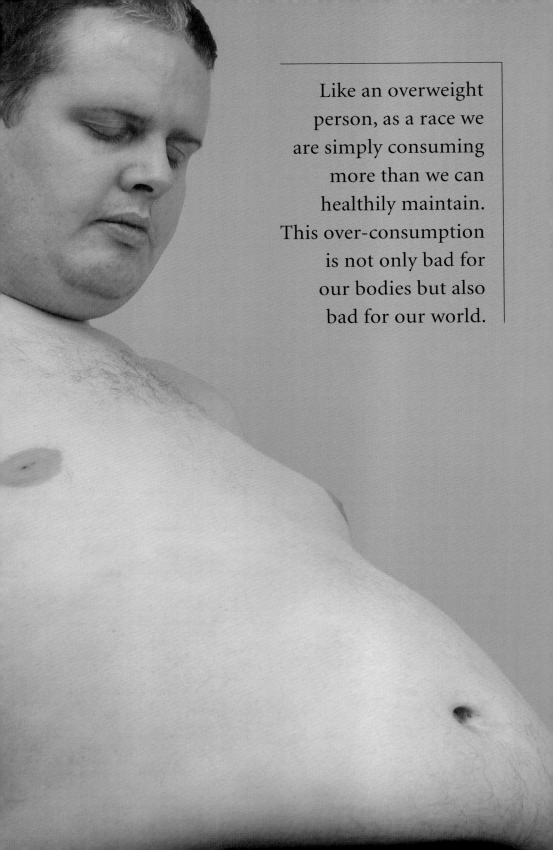

Like an overweight person, as a race we are simply consuming more than we can healthily maintain. This over-consumption is not only bad for our bodies but also bad for our world.

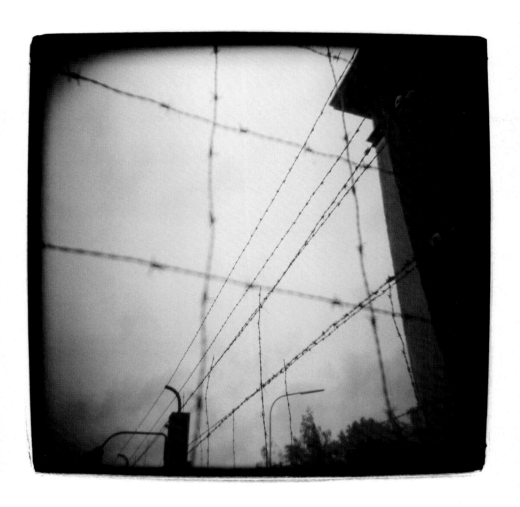

Choose to exercise as an act
of political will. Don't let
yourself become the prisoner
of a collapsing health system,
in which one of the primary
causes of death is poor
medical treatment.

TRAINING FOR LIFE

2nd Floor →

We must learn to look after ourselves better: to exercise daily and to eat food that is healthier for our bodies and the planet.

reported on research conducted at Northwestern University with 3500 arthritis patients. Those who exercised regularly were much less likely to suffer from problems like losing the ability to climb stairs or being unable to bathe or get in and out of bed without assistance.

11. Exercise helps beat depression

Forget the pills. In cases of mild or moderate depression, exercise has been shown to be just as effective as antidepressants — and it's a lot cheaper. Hundreds of studies now show that regular exercise helps relieve anxiety, severe depression and chronic mental illness.

In January 2006, Great Britain's Mental Health Foundation recommended that doctors should be offering all patients with depression a programme of exercise to help combat their malaise.

A November 2005 report from Duke University in Durham, North Carolina reported that just ten minutes of regular, moderate exercise outperformed a leading antidepressant, Zoloft, in easing symptoms in young adults diagnosed with moderate to severe depression. 'Exercise seems to be at least as effective as standard antidepressant medications in reducing symptoms of patients with major depression,' noted the researchers.

Exercise can have a positive effect right away for people who have recently been diagnosed with a major depressive disorder. Researchers at the University of Texas, as reported in the December 2005 issue of *Medicine and Science in Sports and Exercise*, found that those who walked briskly on a treadmill for 30 minutes felt more vigorous and had a greater sense of psychological well-being. The article said that for mildly to moderately depressed patients, exercise could also lessen feelings of isolation and helplessness.

In November 2005, the *Harvard Mental Health Letter* pointed out that there were a large number of studies which showed that exercise could help some people overcome depression.

There's a myriad of possible explanations. People develop an enhanced body image with regular exercise. They get social support in exercise groups. Exercising distracts them from everyday worries, and they develop their self-confidence by meeting goals. Exercise may alter the circulation of neurotransmitters like serotonin, neuropinephrine and, of course, boosts endorphins. You do indeed get a lift from exercise.

12. Exercise helps you to survive bowel cancer

If you're thin and you exercise regularly, then your chances of surviving bowel cancer are higher. In January 2006, *Gut*, an international journal of gastroenterology and hepatology, reported on research from Alfred Hospital in Melbourne. Of 526 people with stage two and stage three bowel cancer, there was a 35 per cent greater chance of survival among those who exercised regularly before diagnosis and had healthy waist measurements (under 94 cm for men or less than 80 cm for women). 'This is a huge reduction [in the death rate],' said Dr Andrew Hayden, leader of the research team. 'We don't see reductions anywhere near this big with chemotherapy. We were surprised by the magnitude of the benefit.'

The Auckland Regional Public Health Service has said that physical activity plays a convincing role in protecting against bowel cancer. Physical activity 'increases insulin sensitivity and thus reduces the levels of circulating insulin, thereby diminishing its effects on tumour development and growth.' Physical activity aids in regular bowel movements and this reduces the time that the colon is exposed to potential carcinogens. It may also alter a number of inflammatory immune factors that influence bowel cancer risks.

13. Exercise saves you money on health care

On average, older Americans who exercise regularly spend $2200 less a year on health care than those who don't exercise, according to a report in the January 2007 issue of the *Lansing State Journal*. The Partnership for Prevention adds that, on average, the annual health care costs for someone with a chronic condition such as diabetes or hypertension — both of which can be helped with a regular exercise regime and a good diet — are five times that of someone who doesn't have such a condition.

14. Exercise helps your back

People have always said that yoga is good for your back and now we have proof. In December 2005, the *Annals of Internal Medicine* published research from a study by the Group Health Cooperative Centre for Health Studies. In it, three groups of patients took part in three different therapies. Those patients who took part in 12-week yoga programme had better back function, and fewer of them used pain relievers.

In California, a 2005 study of 314 patients with chronic back pain conducted at the Spine and Sport Foundation in San Diego showed that an exercise programme of eight to fifteen weeks was more effective in relieving pain and improving functionality than any form of passive treatment.

15. Exercise improves your memory

A University of California at Los Angeles research project presented at the December 2005 annual meeting of the American College of Neuropsychopharmacology showed that a 14-day programme involving regular exercise, stress-reduction exercises and healthy nutrition was found to improve memory in older adults.

A study by researchers at Toulouse University in France, reported in October 2006 in the journal *Neurology*, concluded that overweight middle-aged adults scored more poorly on tests of memory, attention and learning ability than their thinner peers.

16. Exercise helps to prevent prostate cancer

Research conducted by the University of California with a group of approximately 900 men showed that the higher their lean body mass, the lower their risk of prostate cancer. This was especially true of the most aggressive forms of prostate cancer. (As reported in the December 2005 issue of the *Journal of Urology*.)

17. Exercise is good for your career

Recently, *theladders.com*, an online recruiting company for the $100,000+ employment market, reported that of 1000 senior executives in the United States, 75 per cent believed that 'physical fitness is critical for career success at the executive level'. Seventy-five per cent also said that in today's workplace, being overweight is a serious career impediment.

18. Exercise prevents ovarian cancer

As with many cancers, exercise seems to have a preventative effect on ovarian cancer. In one study, women who exercised moderately and more often had a one third lower rate of ovarian cancer than those women who exercised less.

There are several biological mechanisms that explain the protective effect of physical activity on ovarian cancer. Physical activity may mediate levels of endogenous sexual and metabolic hormone and growth factors. Exercise may, through its effect on obesity, decrease the risk by reducing lifetime exposure to endogenous estrogens. Other possible mechanisms include enhancement of the immune system and improvement of the antioxidant defence systems.

19. Exercise is good for your bones

The International Osteoporosis Foundation's 2005 report entitled *Move it or Lose It* notes that weight-bearing and high-impact exercise is best for stimulating bone formation. Dr Helmut Minne — a leading German practitioner who serves on the IOF's board of directors — says: 'Exercise builds strong muscles which in turn build strong bones. Exercise also improves muscle control, balance and co-ordination and reduces the risk of falling or suffering a fracture during a fall.'

The report notes that bone is living tissue that requires weight-bearing and high-impact exercise like dancing, walking, jogging, sports or strength training to stimulate its formation. The new document also highlights a Finnish study that found that physically active young women enter adulthood with 40 per cent more bone mass than sedentary girls of the same age.

20. Exercise is good for your guts

The September 2006 issue of *Clinical Gastroenterology and Hepatology* reports that the number one predictor of abdominal pain, including irritable bowel syndrome, bloating, constipation and diarrhoea, is lack of exercise. Even obese people experience fewer symptoms of irritable bowel syndrome and less gut pain if they exercise, according to the authors of the study.

21. Exercise can prevent strokes

As reported in *Stroke*, a journal of the American Heart Association, research tracking 27,721 Finns aged 25 to 64 over 19 years found that the risk of all forms of stroke among men and women with high levels of physical activity was 26 per cent lower than it was among men and women with low levels of physical activity. The risk of intracerebral haemorrhage was 37 per cent lower for those in the more active group and the risk of sub-arachnoid stroke was 54 per cent lower for those involved in high levels of physical activity.

22. Exercise is good for menopause

Dr Lila Nachtigall, Professor of Obstetrics and Gynaecology at New York University School of Medicine, says that regular exercise is the most effective means of moderating symptoms of menopause including hot flushes, night sweats, sleeplessness and irritability.

23. Exercise is essential for your arteries

This is one of the best-researched areas of exercise benefit. Literally thousands of studies over the past several decades have shown the protective effects of exercise against cardiovascular disease. The American Heart Association sums it up as follows: 'Physical inactivity is a major risk factor for developing coronary artery disease. It also contributes to other risk factors, including obesity, high blood pressure, high triglycerides, a low level of HDL ("good") cholesterol and diabetes. Even moderately intense physical activity such as brisk walking is beneficial when done regularly for a total of 30 minutes or longer on most days.'

A 2005 study at Indiana University, published in the *European Journal of Applied Physiology*, has shown that exercising after a high-fat meal not only reverses damage to arteries, but also improves their function compared to before the meal. Professor Janet P Wallace, co-author of the study, says that for a period of four to six hours after a high-fat meal (i.e. generally just in time for the next meal), our arteries look just like those of a person who has heart disease. The oxidation of high-fat meals causes stress markers that harm the arteries and contribute to heart disease, diabetes, Alzheimer's and cancer. 'What our study showed,' she says, 'is that when you exercise after that meal, it doesn't look like a sick artery anymore.'

● | **PAIN VERSUS PLEASURE**

As human beings we are motivated to change our behaviours for two major reasons. One is the pursuit of pleasure: I want a better house so I'll work overtime. The other is the avoidance of pain: if I don't pay the phone bill, it will be disconnected.

All of the medical evidence tells us that exercising rocks! It's great for us on so many levels. The pleasure of being outdoors, achieving goals, staying healthy, sharing time with friends and family, being part of a club or gym community . . . the list goes on and on. And yet some people just won't take action until they have a major health scare. Their doctor literally petrifies them into action: 'If you don't start exercising, you'll be dead before Christmas.'

While it's never too late, there are no guarantees that you'll recover from a big health issue. If you're not active, get going — now. And if you're already taking care of yourself, we urge you to invite people in your sphere of influence to join you.

More and more studies are published every week highlighting the benefits of exercise. We think it's important that we all understand more about how our bodies work and how best to look after them, for the *entire* duration of the journey.

The following is a more in-depth explanation the science around some of these benefits.

The benefits of strength training

Anti-ageing

Being strong has all sorts of positive effects on our everyday lives. It makes us functionally more efficient — for example, able to pick up our children or carry the shopping more easily, and less likely to injure ourselves in doing so. As we age, this becomes more and more important; maintaining our strength enables us to keep enjoying our lives by comfortably performing daily activities, and protects us from falls and accidents that can send us into life-threatening downward health spirals.

It also increases the density of our bones, which means that we avoid the pains of osteoporosis and that if we do fall, we are less likely to break something. The maxim 'use it or lose it' becomes more and more real.

The good news is that many studies have proved that by exercising to maintain our strength, we are able to maintain optimal function until at least 85 years of age. Even people who have stopped exercising can make tremendous strength gains well into their 90s. A study at Tufts University involving an eight-week strength training programme by women aged 87 to 96 resulted in a tripling of strength and an increase in muscle size of 10 per cent!

Not only does resistance exercise make us function better and protect us from potentially life-shortening injuries, it makes us feel better and *actually age more slowly*. Likely reasons for this are that strength training stimulates the activity of our immune system and the production of many of the hormones responsible for cell regeneration, our normal production of which, as explained earlier, begins to slow down in our early 40s.

Back rehabilitation

Over the years, we and the members of our teams have seen thousands of people rehabilitate themselves from one of the most common physical miseries of post-industrial man — back pain — just by strengthening their backs with simple exercises like the old-fashioned barbell dead-lift. Certain types of weight training and Pilates work, often referred to as core or stability training, are increasingly being used in back rehabilitation in preference to surgery. This commonly involves exercises that are performed using different-sized stability balls, pulleys and other specialised equipment. It is a wonderful new field, administered by specialist trainers and physiotherapists, which is being used by athletes to increase their functional strength and balance; it is also changing people's lives by freeing them from pain and long-term loss of function through surgery.

Clinicians have recently adapted this type of therapy to sophisticated machines like the MedX Core Spinal Fitness System. American readers can find a doctor or therapist practising this and other non-surgical rehab systems at *www.aapmr.org*, the website of the American Academy of Physical Medicine and Rehabilitation.

Most local gyms or personal trainers will be able to give you a programme to strengthen your back and protect yourself against the likelihood of back pain. Just remember that, as stated earlier in this chapter, you have to create joint balance by strengthening opposing muscle groups. In the case of backs, this means strengthening the abdominal muscles as well as the back muscles — especially the lower, deeper abs known as the transverse abdominus and the internal obliques, which stabilise the spine.

With any resistance exercises (even lifting the groceries), the heavier you lift, the more important it becomes to keep your lower abs sucked in and a slight curve in your lower back. This protects you from injury and strengthens these spine-stabilising muscles.

Burning that spare tyre

What isn't so well known about strength training is that it's one of the most powerful long-term ways to burn fat. The reason for this is that it increases the size of the body's fat-burning engine. Simply put, muscle burns fat and the more muscle we have, the more fat we burn.

Fat loss is generally regarded as a result of the difference between the energy you put in and the energy you take out of your system. People often interpret this to mean the amount of calories ingested in the form of food versus the number consumed during exercise. But in reality there's a bit more to it.

Muscle mass and Basal Metabolic Rate (BMR)

Metabolism is all the processes by which the body breaks down food and nutrients to build and maintain itself, and to produce energy. Our metabolic rate determines the rate at which we burn calories. It can be increased or decreased by a few well-known — and a few not so well-known — methods.

One of the best-known techniques for increasing our metabolic rate is simply eating breakfast (we'll talk about this in more detail in Chapter 5). Unfortunately this doesn't mean you can eat all day as a means of maintaining a slim figure! Eating-induced metabolic increases account for only 10 per cent of the calories we burn — about 200 per day for a woman and 250 for a man. We can easily consume more than that with a few snacks, so it's better to stick to just three regular meals per day.

Our *basal metabolic rate* (BMR) is the rate at which our bodies burn energy at rest. This varies from person to person, based on factors like sex, height, weight, age, ambient temperature, stress levels and muscle mass. It is responsible for 70 per cent of the energy burned during the average person's day, and helps explain how we burn 70 calories an hour while we sleep!

There are many websites that allow you to calculate your BMR; we Googled *basal metabolic rate* and entered our data into several. We found that Phillip, as a 1.93m, 52-year-old man weighing 90 kg, has a daily resting consumption of approximately 1900 calories. Jackie, a 1.68m, 47-year-old woman weighing 64 kg, burns around 1350. These are the calories we would burn each day *without exercise.*

The good news here is that it's possible to increase our BMR, and the most powerful means of doing this is to increase our lean muscle mass. Every 500 g of muscle burns approximately 50 calories per day, so we can quite easily achieve significant gains, without having to look like the Incredible Hulk.

Studies have shown that the average person can increase his or her BMR by 15 per cent simply by weightlifting three times a week for 20 minutes. For the average woman, this would mean an extra 300 calories burned per day; for the average man, 375 calories. Five hundred calories equates to half a kg per week in fat loss, so you can see where this is headed.

As noted in Chapter 1, a study of fitness classes by Auckland University's sports science department for Les Mills showed that BodyPump had the lowest immediate calorie-burning effect, but *by far* the highest long-term percentage body-fat loss. Other studies have produced similar findings.

In March 2006, the American Heart Association reported on a survey that had been funded by the National Institute of Health in the United States. In it, women doing strength training twice a week over a sustained period had much lower than expected increases in their abdominal fat. 'Strength training can prevent increases in body fat percentages and alleviate increases in the fat deposit most closely associated with heart disease,' the researchers wrote.

Provided that we don't increase our nutritional intake, a decent weight training programme will increase our net fat loss by up to half a kg per week. Our overall bodyweight won't necessarily change, because the muscle we put on may balance out the fat we shed, but we'll look much trimmer and more toned — and be stronger and healthier, too

---

STRATEGY 14 GET STRONG

Sports like rowing and cycling have high strength components, as do many fitness classes. Weight training, Pilates and yoga provide the most controlled, balanced way to get strong, provided that they're carefully programmed. Strength training

makes us live longer and feel better, and increases our ability to function in sports and in everyday life. It's also the fastest way to look taut, trim and terrific; who honestly doesn't want that?

Optimising your cardio component

For all the benefits of strength training, there are at least as many produced by cardiovascular or 'fitness' exercise. They include lower blood pressure; higher HDL ('good') cholesterol; lower LDL ('bad') cholesterol; decreased glucose-stimulated insulin secretion; improved heart and lung function; decreased stress, anxiety and depression; and, of course, lower body fat. All of these combine to dramatically lower your risk of suffering ailments like heart attacks and strokes. Higher fitness levels also increase your enjoyment of everyday life by giving you more stamina and more energy.

When the research really started coming through on the benefits of exercise, the recommendations were pretty tame . . . three gentle half-hour workouts a week were all that was prescribed. Publicity was given to facts like the conductors on British double-decker buses living several years longer than the drivers. More recent studies, however, suggest that those early recommendations were not enough. To deal with our 21st century Western diet and lifestyle, and to gain optimal benefits, we should be exercising almost every day for up to an hour, at a much higher level of intensity.

The latest American Heart Association guidelines urge all women to exercise for a minimum of 30 minutes per day. Women who need to lose weight or maintain weight loss are now advised to engage in 60 to 90 minutes of moderate-intensity activity on most, or preferably all, days of the week.

The effect of intensity on calorie burning

In addition to the 70 per cent of calories the average person burns as a result of their BMR and the 10 per cent used up as a result of eating, we burn a further 20 per cent through daily exercise activities . . . everything from doing the washing to climbing stairs to simply fidgeting at our desks. This is an average percentage, though, which can be increased to a much higher figure.

At several BMR websites we were able to add our daily exercise quotas to our earlier BMR data and *roughly* calculate our actual daily calorie expenditure or *active metabolic rate* (AMR). In Phillip's case this was around 3300 calories and in Jackie's, approximately 2500. As very active individuals, these equated to 50-85 per cent more than our respective basal or resting metabolic rates. These are rough calculations and we wouldn't recommend doubling your calorie intake based on them, but they give an idea of the huge difference exercise can make to weight maintenance.

Various studies show the body's calorie consumption as a result of different sports and exercise activities ranging from 200 per hour to more than 1000. A study conducted by Auckland University for Les Mills International in 1997 showed calorie burns ranging from 250 to 850 for individuals participating in various Les Mills classes.

It's important to note that your rate of calorie consumption will depend on how much intensity you put in, of course, and as explained above, on other factors like your muscle mass. There's a virtuous circle here — the more exercise you do, especially if there's a strength component, the greater your lean muscle mass and the more calories you will burn as a result of the same amount of exercise! But what is the optimum level of intensity?

Aerobic vs. anaerobic

There's a lot of controversy over the ideal level of exercise intensity for fat burning. Some sources promote the idea that to burn fat you need to work at a low level of intensity. This is based on the theory that, biochemically, the body will burn fat as a primary fuel during low intensity exercise, but not during high intensity exercise.

There are different biochemical means by which our bodies produce the energy required for exercise. This is a very complex subject, but the simple version goes like this:

For very short, explosive bursts of movement, up to around two seconds, our bodies can use stored muscle energy called adenosine triphosphate (ATP). For another three to five seconds we can convert another compound stored in our muscles, creatine phosphate (CP), into ATP. Once the ATP and CP stores are depleted the body resorts to carbohydrate (stored in the blood as glucose and in the muscles and liver as glycogen) as its energy source. At a lower rate of intensity, our body has time to use protein, fats and carbohydrate, combined with oxygen, to produce energy.

Coming at it from the other end, this last energy production system is known as the aerobic system, and is the predominant system used when we exercise for sustained periods of lower intensity exercise such as jogging. When we start to increase the intensity, the second to last system, called the anaerobic system, starts to cut in. It's predominant when we're running, rowing or cycling flat out (or nearly so) for bursts of say 10 seconds to a few minutes. For shorter bursts of strength or explosive activity, such as weightlifting, wrestling or sprinting, the first two systems — collectively called the phosphate energy system — are dominant.

The argument that lower intensity exercise is better for fat-burning is based on the fact that we use fat for fuel only during aerobic energy metabolism. But this doesn't take the whole picture into account. While we don't use fat as a fuel as part of the immediate process of producing energy via the anaerobic and phosphate systems, during most higher-intensity exercise activities we are actually using a combination of all energy systems. The various systems oscillate and interchange as we chase the ball and recover; perform a hard interval followed by an easy one; or just waver back and forwards from our threshold during a run.

phillip It's actually impossible to exercise purely anaerobically for more than about 20–30 seconds. During my sports career I've taken part in lab tests in which I've been required to push to the anaerobic maximum. At the Institute of Sport in Australia they'd put gas analysis masks on us (to precisely measure our fitness) and have us pedal at absolutely top speed on an exercise bike for 60 seconds. After about 25 seconds you'd be completely spent and the last 30 seconds were the longest you'd ever experienced in your life. You'd effectively be blacked out for the last 15 seconds, with your legs barely turning over: they'd have to lift you off the bike and it would take 20 minutes to recover, during which they'd take blood samples every five minutes or so to add to the misery.

More importantly, however, the phosphates and glycogen that we use via the first two systems don't just come out of thin air — they must be replenished *via the aerobic energy system* during recovery (both during and after the workout).

Depending on the intensity and duration of the workout, the replenishment can burn more energy than the exercise did! Anaerobic metabolism is very inefficient. A molecule of glucose produces just two molecules of ATP anaerobically versus up to 36 aerobically. That can mean a whole lot of replenishment during recovery time — either during or after your sports game or fitness class.

Studies measuring what exercise scientists call *excess post-exercise oxygen consumption* (EPOC) have shown that our metabolic rate can be elevated for up to two days after an intense workout, as our bodies replenish their fuel stores, restore hormone balances, and conduct cell repair and growth.

The conclusion here is one that may seem obvious for the lay person, but has been strangely obscure for some experts: the harder you exercise, the more weight you will lose. Think of it like this: there aren't many fat sprinters. There is also plenty of evidence of higher intensity exercise, within limits, having a greater positive effect on our ageing, our immune system and our health.

Finding balance

Exercise at a lower level, however, is still likely to give you benefits, and there are other great arguments for it. For most people, for instance, it is simply more palatable and therefore more likely to keep us active. While elite athletes may be prepared to put themselves through gruelling workouts in pursuit of Olympic glory, too much pain will scare most of us off.

We can find ways to disguise the pain; fun ways of exercising harder, like those described in Chapter 3. But even then there are physical limits to the amount of work we can absorb.

We get the maximum benefit when we work out fresh and are able to give it maximum effort. But most of us can only put our bodies through a couple of very tough workouts a week. After that we start to suffer the effects of overtraining, as we discussed in Chapter 1: diminishing returns and an increased risk of injury.

To maintain optimum health we need to work out almost every day. This means balancing our training cycle throughout the week with hard, medium and easy days as well as varied activities (see cross-training, Chapter 1) that allow us to optimise our programme.

● | **SUMMARY OF PART ONE: ENERGY OUT**

At the end of the day, we need to find the ways that individually suit us to get as much exercise into our lives as we can. Choosing to exercise, and getting ourselves into great shape, is important on a micro and a macro scale. Living an active life will keep us healthier and happier, for longer. Our families will benefit and we'll set a good example for our children. But there's more to it than that. Being fit and healthy is becoming an act of social responsibility.

Federal forecasters in the US have conservatively predicted that by 2016 the cost of the American health system will have doubled to $4.1 trillion dollars per year. With 75 per cent of this expenditure already going to the treatment of chronic illness, a huge percentage of this increase will be the result of inactive aging and obesity-based disease. Imagine how much more effectively we could spend any portion of that increase rather than on treating ourselves for preventable illnesses stemming from inactivity and excessive consumption.

Just a tiny fraction of that increase, $40–$60 billion a year, is the estimated additional foreign aid required to achieve the 2015 UN Millennium Development Goals, according to OECD figures. Those goals include:

- cutting in half extreme poverty and hunger

- achieving universal primary education

- eliminating gender disparity at all levels of education

- reducing the under-five mortality rate by two thirds

- reducing the maternal mortality rate by three quarters

- reversing the spread of HIV/AIDS

- cutting the proportion of people without access to clean water in half

- significantly improving the lives of at least 100 million slum dwellers.

PricewaterhouseCoopers estimates that we could reduce carbon emissions sufficiently to stave off the effects of global warming by spending two to three percent of world GDP by 2050, i.e. by spending around one trillion a year in today's dollars; half the projected 2006–16 increase in US health costs.

Choose to exercise as a way of ensuring the survival of our planet. Ride a bike, instead of being sole navigator on a suburban safari in your SUV.

Choose to exercise as an act of political will. Don't let yourself become the prisoner of a collapsing health system, in which one of the primary causes of death is poor medical treatment.

If you believe in a higher being, exercise because your designer came up with a wonderful body for your spirit to live in and you should look after it.

If you're an atheist, choose to exercise because it will help determine the kind of world you pass on to your children and your grandchildren.

And if you're overweight and feeling as though it's all too hard and you've left it too late, take comfort from the knowledge that we know thousands of people all over the globe who have found the courage to get started. Find hope in their stories and be encouraged by their success. We hope that some of the tools and techniques discussed in this part of the book will help you begin and continue your fitness journey.

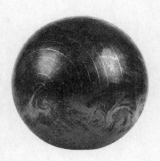

part two | energy in

Like an overweight individual, as a race we are simply consuming far more than we can healthily maintain. This overconsumption is bad for our bodies and bad for our world. Eating less (which means eating smarter) and supporting the sustainable-organic movement will not only do a huge amount of good for our personal health, but also help preserve the planet.

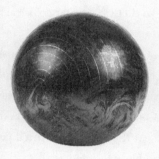

5 | downsize me

As we said in Chapter 3, this is a game of inches, both literally and figuratively. The vast majority of people do not go on a 'super-size me' diet at McDonald's like the maker of the famous documentary film. Most of us simply put on one or two pounds (up to a kg) a year from around the age of 20, until by the age of 40 we are 20-40 pounds (9–18 kg) overweight. *The average person never loses the weight they put on after eating Christmas dinner.*

There's no easy cure. It's virtually impossible to lose weight quickly — for both physiological and psychological reasons. Our bodies are amazing, complex machines that operate instinctively: when was the last time you had to remind yourself to breathe? That's why traditional diets don't work. If you go on a starvation diet your body goes into primal famine-response mode. It panics and, thinking that food supplies are running out, it slows down your metabolism — which slows your body's calorie consumption. Faster than you can say chocolate-coated doughnut, your body actually starts *preserving* fat stores. Rather than getting rid of fat, your body will consume bone, muscle, organ tissue — anything, in fact, other than brain tissue — before it will consume fat in what it perceives to be a starvation situation. We evolved this system to help us to survive long periods without food in our ancient past. Fantastic these days if you're lost in the bush for a week, but terrible if you're trying to lose weight.

Then, traditional theory goes, when we do finally lose some fat, most of us give up the diet and the legacy of our primal starvation-response kicks in. Our fat cells gobble up even more than they did before. In effect, we actually re-train our fat cells. If we start yo-yo dieting, our fat cells learn to absorb more — just in case we're thinking of starving them again.

A newer explanation for the phenomenon of post-dietary fat gain is that each time we diet, we lose muscle as well as fat. It's more difficult to put muscle back on than fat, so with each diet our muscle mass decreases and, with it, our basal metabolic rate. One way or another, diets that involve losing lots of weight rapidly, usually defeat their purpose. You'll get fatter in between diets than you would have if you hadn't dieted at all.

Psychologically as well, it's very difficult to make and maintain the drastic changes that crash diets require. Ordinary human frailties, combined with guilt associated with failure to stick to strict diet rules, can lead to further overeating and create a miserable, self-defeating cycle.

The most successful dietary changes are the ones that are made by gradually removing over-nutrition, and creating an eating pattern that gives us enough energy to live healthy lives and steadily decrease — or at least not increase — our weight over a period of years. If you want to be significantly slimmer for the rest of your life, then all the research shows you must find a way to incorporate exercise into your life. However, intelligent eating alone can stop you from becoming obese — and it will certainly assist your exercise programme.

500 a day keeps the doctor away

In pure nutritional terms, if we reduce our calorie intake by 500 calories a day we can lose 500 g a week, which is within the healthy weight-loss limits recommended by most authorities. We have to be careful here, as this depends on what our calorie intake currently is. If you're already on 1200–1500 calories a day, which is at the bottom of the recommended range for sedentary women, and you reduce that by 500 calories, you're going to be on a dangerously low intake. You'll certainly put yourself into primal famine-response mode, and you may put your health at risk as well.

The UK Health Department's estimated daily requirements are 1940 calories for the average woman and 2550 for the average man. A low calorie diet is defined as 800–1200 calories per day (800–1500 by some experts); very low is 600–800. All of these figures actually vary from person to person depending on activity levels and basal metabolic rates — which are in turn based on sex, height, weight, age and muscle mass. However, most diets below 1200 calories a day don't contain enough essential nutrients for long-term health. Diets below 800 should only be followed when obesity is creating an immediate medical danger. Anyone eating so few calories requires close medical supervision. There are major risks involved, including organ damage and failure.

On the other hand, if you're somebody who is eating thousands of calories a day and exercising little, then a 500 calorie per day reduction may work for you — not by crash dieting, but by gradually reducing your intake, particularly of high-fat and high-energy foods.

Five hundred fewer calories a day might not sound like a lot — just a few chocolate biscuits — but it's something most of us find remarkably difficult.

In this chapter we highlight a number of techniques that have proved to be the most successful long-term approaches in the weight-loss industry in recent years, plus a few personal ones of our own.

Don't try to use them all at once. Instead, set yourself a goal of incorporating one or two techniques into your lifestyle every few weeks. Start with the ones that seem easiest to you. Then, as you successfully incorporate them into your daily life, add another one or two. It's a game of inches.

Appendix 1 contains a quick summary list that you can cut out and stick on your refrigerator as a reminder, or to check off as you successfully adopt each technique. You can also download and print a copy of this at *www.lesmills.com*.

Don't buy junk with your weekly shopping

This is a remarkably simple — and effective — technique. People consume most of their calorie intake at home, so shop carefully. Go shopping after you've had a meal or have something light beforehand: avoid visiting the supermarket when you're hungry.

Don't buy any sweets, soft drinks or sodas, biscuits, cakes, snack bars, ice cream, potato chips, crisps or chocolate. Even when they're on special.

If we set our minds to it, most of us are able to find the discipline to control our impulses during a half-hour shopping trip. Very few of us are able to maintain that discipline for 168 hours a week once the junk food is in the house. If you don't buy it and it's not in the cupboards, you're much less likely to eat it. Period.

Don't take your kids shopping

We don't mean to sound bombastic here. A lot of parents find it hard to resist their kids' demands. That's because it *is* hard. It's very difficult when you're a parent and you're short on time and sleep, and the kids are constantly haranguing you about this and that. It's virtually impossible to stand up to their nagging at the supermarket when they're dead-set on sweets.

One way around this is to make it a rule that you don't take your kids shopping. Leave them at home with your partner, or do the shopping while they're at school or childcare. How many times have you seen a stressed-out parent with a whining child wanting a chocolate bar on a winter's night in the supermarket queue? Have you ever noticed how the snacks aimed at kids are at eye level for them?

Kids will break you down. You're tired, you're busy and you've got a thousand other things to think about. They've got one thing to think about: getting that treat they want *right now*. They are superb at wearing us down and getting their own way. So don't take the little devils shopping.

jackie | Sometimes we just don't have a choice about whether or not to take our kids. A policy that my sisters and I adopted for those situations was to allow them to select one thing only. It was wonderfully involving for the kids and became their weekly treat!

Don't buy soft drinks and sodas

We mentioned soft drinks/sodas under junk food, but they do deserve their own section. They're pure poison. Don't even consider letting your kids drink them. Ever.

Don't buy fruit juice

We're still on the things to leave out of your trolley. It breaks our heart to say this about fruit juice, as many freshly squeezed organic juices obviously don't fall into the junk food category. But for most of us, they are nevertheless better left at the supermarket. Why? A glass of apple or orange juice (236–335 ml) normally contains 100–200 calories, whereas an orange or an apple normally contains a third to a half of that. Juice is also terrible for kids' teeth because of the amount of sugar it contains and its acidity. Never put it in a baby's drinking bottle or drinking cup. Dentists these days are seeing a lot of children with rotten teeth and a growing percentage of kids are having their first set of teeth removed. The major reason for this is juice and soft drinks/sodas. It seems all right in the short term because it's only their first set of teeth, but the second set of teeth then grow unevenly and can necessitate orthodontics in the kids' teenage years.

We're not saying that you shouldn't buy yourself and your kids a fresh fruit and vegetable juice in place of junk food when you're at the mall; just don't have it at home. As we've said, it is easy to discipline yourself for 30 minutes or so when you're in the store, but it's difficult not to drink it when it's in the house. If you've been a juice addict, you and other members of the household will quickly rediscover the wonderful taste of water when you remove the other options.

STRATEGY 15 DON'T PICK UP JUNK FOOD WHEN YOU BUY THE GROCERIES

This includes cakes, cookies/biscuits, chocolate, deep-fried anything, candy, sweets, high-energy muesli bars, fizzy drinks, sodas, potato chips, pretzels . . . you get the idea. Keep it out of the trolley, out of your cupboards, out of your hands, out of your mouth and out of your body.

jackie We make fresh organic fruit and vegetable juice at home three times a week, as a way to increase our intake of beta-carotenoids and other nutrients essential to a truly healthy diet. It's also a marvellous way to help adolescent skin. If you can buy a juicer, the combination of carrot and apple plus anything else the family will drink are perfect. We have this in place of dessert.)

Eat three correctly sized meals a day

These days, most people know not to skip breakfast and lunch because of the effect it has on slowing down metabolism and, in turn, actually slowing down the body's rate of energy consumption. Think back to the starvation responses we talked about at the beginning of this chapter. Give your body a break. Eat breakfast and lunch every day so that your body knows that all is well in your world. Your metabolism will work properly if you feed it great food at regular intervals.

In our experience, however, eating many small meals a day doesn't tend to work, unless you're an elite athlete training for hours and hours a day. It's OK in principle — it keeps the metabolism from slowing — but in fact this effect, known as *dietary thermogenisis*, is only responsible for about ten per cent of the average person's daily calorie consumption. (The vast majority comes from basal metabolic rate and physical activity.) The positive effect we can create by eating many meals is outweighed, for most of us, by the fact that we lack the discipline to restrict the size of the meals.

A diet of five or six small meals a day tends to result in our taking in more calories; also, we can develop a habit of always thinking about food and what we're going to eat next.

Serve smaller portions

Don't feel as though you have to serve yourself and your family huge portions to keep them satisfied. We've got to get over the habit of thinking that food is a way to our family's hearts — or, rather, that *lots* of food is a way to our family's hearts.

The 'bigger is better' mentality was a sign of prosperity after the Depression, and of stability after the two world wars. It was a way of showing that everything worked, that we were a better society, but it has now turned around to bite us. It's created huge environmental problems that we talk about in the next chapter — and it's making us fat. (This does not just affect developed countries. In India, as in Western countries in earlier times, being overweight is a sign of being prosperous and middle class and is therefore desirable. This attitude is helping to create a growing problem with type 2 diabetes there.) We have to change this mentality.

Personal trainer Jac Falloon, who we mentioned in Chapter 2, tells an insightful story about one of her clients:

> Sally had been working with me for weeks; her goal was to lose eight kg in time for her sister's wedding, where she was going to be Matron of Honour. I designed a nutrition and exercise plan for her and initially things went really well, but then we hit a plateau where Sally just didn't seem to be able to lose any more weight. She insisted that she was following my menu plans, which listed the types of food to eat each day. I was stumped.
>
> A week or so later Sally invited me to her birthday dinner and I enjoyed a lovely, healthy, low-fat meal that Sally had prepared for me and two other friends, and after dessert I left. Well, ten minutes later my cellphone rang and it was Sally, in tears. 'Now I understand,' she said. 'I saw how much — or rather how little — you had on the plate and so that's all I had too. But I spent the whole night thinking about the fact that I would normally have taken at least twice as much food.'

Sally was in the habit of serving herself massive portions and then eating the leftovers as she cleared up. Even though the food was healthy and low fat, she was simply eating way too much of it.

In the 21st century we need to move towards the idea that small is beautiful. We have to starting choosing smaller cars, smaller houses and, of course, less to eat.

One simple way to achieve this is to put smaller portions on your plate. If it's there, you'll eat it. If it's not, you won't. A variation is to consciously cook less food. Measure the ingredients you use in your favourite dishes and reduce them by one third to a half.

You can also try smaller plates. They look full with less food on them. This might seem cute, but it works. All of the food for your meal — including the entrée that you're eating separately if you're having one — should fit on a medium-sized plate. It if doesn't, you're probably eating too much. Invest in a dinner set that will help you eat less. It can be that simple.

Don't prepare multi-course meals

Having smaller portions is not an excuse to prepare multi-course meals. You know the sensation of feeling full after the main course at a restaurant but always having more room for dessert? That's because we can satiate our hunger for one type of food but still crave another. The easiest way around that, at a restaurant or at home, is to have just one course.

Learn to make a great salad

If you must have more than one course, then start with a salad. This was found to be one of the keys to the success of the heart-friendly Mediterranean diet, which was mentioned in Chapter 4. You satiate your initial hunger and the high fluid and fibre content of the vegetables makes you feel full, so you eat less of the high-energy food in the main course.

We like to mix a variety of salad greens, tomatoes and cucumbers with roasted sunflower seeds and a little aged balsamic vinegar for dressing. If that's too sparse for you, dress it with a few drops of light vinaigrette made from good olive oil and vinegar. (Olive oil is a healthy unsaturated fat, but it is relatively high calorie.) Better still, have a salad as your entire meal. We often throw in some goat cheese and/or tempeh for protein and leave it at that.

For recipes that are simply wonderful for salads (and just about everything else), we recommend *The Moosewood Cookbook* by Mollie Katzen, *Rock Around The Kitchen* by Madonna's old chef Peter Chaplin and Mary Cox, and *The Healthy Kitchen* by Dr Andrew Weil and ex-Oprah chef Rosie Daley. These authors all really understand nutrition and how to eat in a way that's delicious — and good for the planet.

Learn how to make a tasty, nutritious salad and you'll change the pattern of your eating. You can make this healthy option a favourite for your family. Just don't put sugar in the dressing

When eating out, just order an appetiser

While eating at many different restaurants around the world, one of the alarming things we have noticed is the size of portions in the US. American portion sizes are — and this is common knowledge to anyone who travels a lot — much bigger than in other parts of the world, especially southern Europe. The size of these servings is one reason why Americans are leading the obesity epidemic. The US market now needs to reject this trend.

You can control what happens at home, but you can't always control what happens in a restaurant. Many of the great restaurants of the world these days serve multiple courses, but very small portions of each one. So you get the great taste but not the calories.

In 2004 we ate at El Bulli, in the north of Spain, which pioneered 'molecular gastronomy' and was rated by *Restaurant Magazine* as the best restaurant in the world in 2006. Ferran Adrià and his team of 23 chefs spend six months of the year 'in the lab' in Barcelona creating the next season's menu, and open the restaurant for the other six months. It takes years to get a reservation. You are served a 28-course meal but the courses are very small; some of them are literally just foam. You get to the end having experienced a fabulous panorama of tastes, but without feeling bloated.

Obviously you can't go to El Bulli every time you eat out, so ask for entrée-sized — or, in the US, appetiser-sized — portions at restaurants. If a restaurant does serve you oversized portions, don't feel guilty about leaving half of the meal behind.

Personally, we seem to have a lot of guilt associated with food, which we think comes from our parents' insistence that we clean our plates because 'children are starving in Africa'. The parents of baby boomers went through the Depression, as well as one or both world wars, and back then wasting food was a sin.

Now, it's the reverse. In the 1950s, parents still worried about being able to put enough food on their children's plates. We have a different set of circumstances: an over-abundance of food and, in particular, an over-abundance of the calorie-rich food that was once very scarce.

We now need to train ourselves to serve smaller portions and until the restaurants of the world get the message, we should make a virtue of leaving food on our plates.

STRATEGY 16 EAT LESS, THREE TIMES PER DAY

Little tricks like smaller plates, single-course meals and ordering only an appetiser will help you to achieve this. Learn to make good salads and serve smaller portions of great-quality food.

If you're overweight, don't let your family get that way

If you are the member of the household with the weight problem, don't pass it on to your partner, your children or your flatmates. Start to change your shopping habits now.

It's especially important with children: the eating habits they develop as they're growing up will affect them for the rest of their lives. They may complain at first if you begin buying different food, but they won't love you any less for it. In fact, they'll love you more in the long term if you show concern for them.

As we said earlier, keep plenty of fruit and vegetables on hand, as well as organic wholegrain bread for sandwiches or toast. Their taste buds will soon adjust. And if you've still got babies, start them on healthy options from the moment they start on solids and they won't know what they're missing.

Have healthy snacks on hand

It's better to restrict yourself to three well-balanced meals a day, but active kids often need snacks to keep up with their energy demands. It's important to choose the right ones for them — and for you, if you must also snack. Unfortunately, many so-called 'healthy' options are not all they're cracked up to be. Sure, they're sometimes low in fat, but many are packed with energy in the form of sugar and syrups, so if you're trying to reduce your calorie intake you need to avoid these types of bars and nibbles.

As a parent, one easy way to improve your family's diet is to develop some creative, healthy snacks that the whole family will enjoy.

If your kids have already been trained to like junk food, there will be an adjustment period. They'll complain like crazy about it, but rest assured that your kids are in no danger of starving. Ask yourself if you can justify jeopardising their long-term health by giving them unhealthy food.

Don't worry if your kids go through phases where it seems they hardly eat anything. There are times when they won't have a big appetite for months on end. When they need food for a growth spurt, they'll start eating more.

Change your buying habits so your pantry has great snacks for you and your kids. Keep plenty of fruit and vegetables around the house. Sliced apples and oranges are great; because of their high fibre and water content they fill you up quickly, relative to their calorie content. Buy bags of baby organic carrots if they're available, or slice carrot sticks to munch on: they're sweet and juicy and they're filling. You can eat virtually unlimited amounts of most vegetables, apart from the starchy ones like potatoes, without dramatically affecting your calorie count. (A medium-sized tomato has just 15 calories, a large carrot around 50.)

We buy a variety of organic wheat and non-wheat breads for sandwiches or toast. An average slice of wholemeal bread contains 65 calories. We love low-calorie accompaniments like tomatoes and herb salt on toast. We also use tasty olive oils, organic nut butters and unsweetened organic jams, but be careful here; these foods are high calorie and should be drizzled or thinly spread. Experiment a bit. Hummus is a great slightly lower-calorie option (than oils and butters) to have on wholegrain toast, as are bananas and avocados, or sardines if you have a taste for them.

See Table 1 (page 126) for ideas on low-calorie nutritious snacks.

Make healthy food fun

Many of you will already have wised up to the strain our kids are under from advertising and peer pressure. In your own small way, you can take on the giants of the junk food industry by making healthy food fun for you and your kids.

Snack foods and junk foods have been developed to hook kids. They've been engineered with massive amounts of sugar, fat and salt. They're brightly coloured and they're cute: think of the crackers and cheese in one little packet.

You can do all those sorts of things yourself, in a healthy way, using little

TABLE 1 HEALTHY SNACKS

Any type of fruit

Fruit salad topped with natural low-fat yoghurt

1 cup of skim milk served hot or cold (optional: add 1 tsp cocoa*)

Home-made popcorn, especially with a little brewer's yeast

Handful of peanuts or pistachios in their shells (taking off the shells slows you down, making you eat fewer)

Carrot and celery sticks with or without hummus dip

Wholegrain or sourdough toast with sliced banana

Sliced pear or apple and a small chunk of reduced-fat cheese

Smoothie made with 1 cup of low-fat milk, 2 tbsp natural yoghurt and whatever fruit you have; frozen berries are delicious in a smoothie and are packed with antioxidants

Brown rice cakes with 1 tbsp of almond butter or tomato and cracked pepper

Low-fat yoghurt topped with pieces of fruit and 1 tbsp of mixed nuts and seeds

Banana and a glass of low-fat milk

Cup of vegetable soup (this is a great way to increase your veggie intake), without added cream, of course

1 cup of flavoured rice milk

Low-fat fruit yoghurt

Small handful of mixed organic nuts or try tamari roasted almonds. Go easy on peanuts!

Oatcakes topped with banana or reduced-fat cheese

Several dried apricots, figs or prunes

Vegetable juice (lower in energy than fruit juice)

Wholegrain crackers with low-fat cream cheese

Low-fat yoghurt drink

Low-fat rice pudding snack

Slice of toast with avocado and sliced tomato

Slice of fruit toast with low-fat cream cheese

---

* Cocoa has no added sugar and is therefore a better option than drinking chocolate. It is less sweet but you will soon get used to it and will then find drinking chocolate way too sweet.

tricks like cutting kids' sandwiches into cute shapes. You can be creative with how you serve kids' food and how you ensure it's attractive. Make seeds, nuts and dried apricots into treats; emphasise how delicious they are and what fun it is to eat such yummy food.

A dear friend of ours, Sacha Coburn, makes a daily fuss of serving her two kids, aged five and 18 months, a vegetable entrée. She steams three veges every night, alternating between fresh organic and frozen ones from the supermarket. She serves the kids as if she were their waiter in a fine restaurant and makes up silly names for the dishes. 'Mademoiselle, here is your asparagus apparition and for you, sir, parsimonious peas with brontosaurial broccoli.' The kids love it and they only get their 'main' course of protein and carbohydrate when their 'appetizer' is just about all eaten. Sacha says five-year-old Tiger really believes that broccoli is what brontosauruses lived on; she'll try to keep him believing that until he's 23 if that's what it takes!

Let's not fool ourselves that kids are the only suckers for great packaging and convenient, well-marketed foods. Challenge yourself to see past the sizzle and assess the nutritional worth of what you put into your trolley — and, ultimately, into your body.

Learn to make a great soup

At our house we do fabulous soups and salads. We talked about the salads earlier, and soups are another great way to get healthy foods into you and your family. A blender and a little seasoning can transform the most despised vegetables into a mouth-watering, low-calorie delight, and the leftovers can provide a filling snack during the day. The three books we mentioned earlier — *The Moosewood Cookbook, Rock Around The Kitchen* and *The Healthy Kitchen* — contain soup recipes that can literally change your life.

Drink water

When you feel hungry between meals, have a glass of water. It's possible that your body is actually craving fluids and it's telling you to eat as a way of hydrating itself.

If you're a person who's always on the move, squeeze-top bottles are easy to carry around with you and serve as a great visual reminder that cutting back on calories is part of a cleansing process in which you are ridding your body of fat it doesn't need and can't use. Generally, however, it's better to drink filtered water from a tap, for several reasons.

Firstly, there are the ecological problems associated with drink bottles; the plastic ones are oil-based, and with only about 20 per cent of plastic currently being recycled, they add to our waste-disposal problems (see Chapter 10).

Secondly, consider the potential health risks. While the type 1 and 2 plastics (PET and HDPE) most commonly used in drink bottles are currently regarded as safe, we seem to be finding out more and more about the dangers of plastic as time goes on. Types 3, 6 and 7 (PVC, polystyrene and polycarbonate — which is often used in babies' bottles!) have been found to be highly toxic. If you have reusable metal or glass bottles they are probably better, but you must keep them very clean.

Sparkling mineral water at restaurants is OK. The bottles it comes in are normally glass rather than plastic and it's a healthy alternative to higher-calorie drinks.

STRATEGY 17 IF YOU'RE OVERWEIGHT, DON'T LET YOUR FAMILY AND FLATMATES GET THAT WAY

Have a range of healthy snacks at home. This includes fruit, veges, low-fat yoghurts and low-fat cheeses. Drink lots of water and learn to make life-changing soups!

Learn to balance your plate

At our New Zealand gyms we offer a weight-loss programme called BodyRevolution. It combines nutritional advice from one of the world's top nutritionists, Australian Dr Joanna McMillan-Price, with exercise assistance from personal trainers. The results our club members get with this programme are outstanding.

In Appendix 2 we've included the energy-level charts we use to help people determine what to put on their plates. The charts are easy to use. Just find the energy level that best fits your current weight and then read along the chart to find out how many 'blocks' of carbohydrate, protein and fats you should eat every day. You do need to think about your daily menu in advance, but if that seems too much like hard work you can go to *www.lesmills.com* and download weekly meal planners.

We have a nutritionist friend who likens balancing your diet to getting dressed. Most of us learn at an early age which combinations of clothing work and how to dress for our body type. It's the same with food, except that lots of us learn the wrong ways to eat — either from our parents or from the masses of advertising that we're exposed to on a daily basis. She reminds her clients that they wouldn't dream of wearing a short, tight miniskirt over the top of a long, flowing skirt — yet they don't think twice about having a ham and cheese sandwich. Where's the balance? Ham and cheese is protein plus protein. And both are often high in fat. She challenges her clients to educate themselves so that eating great combinations comes as naturally as wearing the perfect outfit.

To achieve healthy and long-term weight loss you need to eat a mix of smart carbohydrates, lean proteins and good fats, heaps of fruit and veges, and lots of water. It's all about balancing what you eat from each of the food groups and making sure that you're consuming the very best nutrients that each group has to offer. Forget the diets that tell you to cut out entire food groups: research has repeatedly shown us that the more extreme a diet is, the harder it is to stick to in the long term and the harder it therefore is to achieve successful lifelong control of your weight. Each food group provides different essential nutrients; the more diverse your diet, the healthier it is likely to be.

There is indeed growing evidence in support of higher protein diets, but this needn't be at the expense of good-quality carbohydrates. If regular exercise is going to be a part of your life, you'll need those carbs in order to give your best at each workout. BodyRevolution advocates that you get 45–50 per cent of your energy intake from carbohydrates, 20–25 per cent from protein and 25–30 per cent from fat, and that you aim to achieve this balance in *every* meal you eat. For most people, this means a reduction in fat and carbohydrates and an increase in protein. But even within this, there are a few tricks you should know . . .

Use good fats

Yes, fat is good for you — if it's the right kind of fat, eaten in sensible quantities. Fats have all sorts of essential health benefits (see Chapter 7). It's also been shown that people on a healthy diet including fats enjoy it more than people on a low-fat diet; they consequently stick with it and lose more weight.

The latest studies indicate that unsaturated fats are more readily used as fuel by the body and are less likely to be stored than saturated fats. Fortunately, this is in line with heart disease research, which also favours unsaturated fats over saturated fats. Transfats found in processed foods are the worst and should be avoided (look for hydrogenated fat/oil in the ingredients list).

Unsaturated fats can be further divided into two families: the omega-3 fats and the omega-6 fats. The ratio of these two groups seems to be particularly important. In the past we would have eaten far more omega-3 and less omega-6 than we do today. For the benefit of our health as well as our figures, we need to redress this balance. This means eating fish and seafood as often as we can, and limiting our use of certain fats and oils. In short:

- reduce your intake of saturated fat — that means less butter, animal fat, dairy fat and most cakes, doughnuts, biscuits and pastries. Ideally, just cut the latter group out altogether

- avoid trans-fats found in processed foods and fried fast foods

- choose a monounsaturated fat as your main oil at home. Olive oil is perfect, but also look for avocado oil, camellia tea oil or nut oils

- eat more fish, especially oily fish, and seafood (if you are worried about mercury levels, simply choose smaller fish lower down the food chain to be sure of reduced levels)

- eat more leafy green plant foods, linseed (sometimes called flaxseed) and lean game meats to further boost omega-3 fat levels.

Unsaturated fats are liquid at room temperature: think of olive oil and seed oils. Table 2 has a list of fats that can do you a lot of good. They include omega-3 fats, which improve brain function and reduce the risk of heart attacks and strokes.

TABLE 2 HEALTHY FATS — CHOOSE MORE OFTEN

Major sources of unsaturated fats:

Olives and olive oil

Avocados

Peanuts and almonds, including their oil and butter

Linseed, canola and mustard seed oils

Other nuts and seeds, including their oils and butters

Major sources of omega-3 unsaturated fats:

Oily fish e.g. salmon (wild rather than farmed), trout, sardines, tuna, herring, anchovies, mackerel

Omega 3-enriched eggs

Note: Avoid hydrogenated versions of any of these fats

Choose low-fat 'real' food options

Many people know this but it's worth repeating, especially given the current propensity for reducing carbs in preference to fat: the bottom line is that high-fat foods have a high energy density. This means we must eat far less of them if we hope to control our weight. Choosing high-fat foods also makes it difficult to control how much we are consuming and we tend to eat more.

The reason low-fat diets that don't appear to have 'worked' for so many of us is that the food industry responded to our requests for low-fat food by producing a plethora of highly processed, albeit low-fat, products in which the fat was replaced by sugars, syrups and other sweeteners. This meant less fat but *not* less energy. We do not advocate these products at all — in fact you should examine carefully anything that says 'diet' on the packet! Instead, choose low-fat 'real' foods: i.e. food as close to its natural state as possible. Think fresh vegetables and fruit, lean meats, fish, seafood and legumes. Then add small quantities of the healthy fats — nuts, seeds, eggs, oily fish, avocado, olive oil — to provide taste and the essential nutrients we need.

Concentrate on reducing saturated fats, and when eating animal and dairy foods substitute low- or non-fat options for full-fat ones wherever possible. Low-fat milk, butter, yoghurt, cheese etc may taste strange at first, but after a few weeks they'll seem normal and the higher-fat ones will begin to taste disgusting. If you're a meat eater, cut off any visible fat before cooking.

Get smart about smart carbs

This is just so important. Many of the recent myths about dieting surround carbohydrates. Low-carb diets and rules like no carbs after 8 pm have been accepted as gospel. This is quite wrong.

Carbohydrates are an essential fuel for exercise; people with low carb stores suffer from fatigue and low energy. Certain carbohydrate-rich foods also contain vital nutrients that reduce our risk of getting cancer, heart disease and all sorts of other illness.

Smart carbs are the more traditional, less processed carbohydrate-rich foods, such as wholegrains, fruit and vegetables. In addition to health and energy-related benefits, they provide a slow, steady release of energy rather than the quick hit that we get from processed carbs in foods such as cakes and cereal bars.

Don't be fooled by the sugar content of foods. Many starchy foods we used to call *complex* carbs (and were advised to eat more of), such as white bread, bagels, potatoes and the majority of processed breakfast cereals, are absorbed much more quickly than unprocessed foods containing sugar. This causes a rapid rise in blood glucose, which stimulates a hormonal response that tells our bodies to store fat. That's then followed by a blood glucose crash that drives us to eat again.

Choose low-GI foods

The glycaemic index (GI) is a ranking of foods containing carbohydrates, based on their measured effect on our blood glucose levels. Table 3 lists some smart carb options, based on the index. All the smart carbs we've listed for you have low GI scores so you'll get the benefits of improved fat loss, as well a reduced risk of diabetes and heart disease.

Of course, the GI is not the be-all and end-all. Some have criticised the index on the basis that many clearly unhealthy food choices have low GI. But it's not intended to be used in isolation. We still have to think about the fat content of foods and the type of fat they contain. For example, ice cream has a low GI but eating gallons of the stuff will clearly not help us to lose weight. Instead, use the GI to be discerning about which carbs you eat, having already selected foods low in saturated (and trans-) fat. In essence these are the minimally processed, more traditional foods.

For more information on the GI go to *www.glycemicindex.com,* where you can search the database for all foods tested and listed on the international tables.

TABLE 3 SMART CARB OPTIONS — CHOOSE MORE OFTEN

Roasted vegetable salads, e.g. carrot, kumara, pumpkin with garlic cloves

Fresh or frozen fruit

Canned fruit in natural juice

Dried apricots or sultanas

Wholegrain bread — look for lots of visible grains

Sourdough bread — even better if also wholegrain or rye

Fruit loaf — with lots of dried fruit and less flour

Muesli (but skip those with added fat and/or sugars);
  All Bran varieties; rolled oats

Brown or basmati rice (but watch quantities). NB: Not all brown rice has a
  low GI, but it generally provides more nutrients than white rice

Bulgur (cracked wheat), quinoa, buckwheat and more 'unusual' grains

Lentils, beans or chickpeas

Traditional durum wheat pasta (but watch quantities). Wholegrain varieties
  have added nutrients and fibre

Barley

Choose protein that packs a punch

There is good evidence that consuming more protein in our diet can help us to lose weight and keep it off. By making sure we eat enough protein at each meal, and cutting down on unhealthy fats and processed, high-GI carbs, we can help our bodies to burn fat.

Protein helps in a number of ways. Firstly, it is very satiating. It makes us feel full and that means that we can eat less of it and still feel as though we've had a good meal. Secondly, it won't produce a rush of sugar followed by a crash that leaves us craving more food shortly afterwards. This helps to keep us feeling satisfied until the next meal, making it less likely that we feel like we need to snack. Thirdly, it's a vital support for any exercise programme, enabling us to recover and build muscle. Studies have shown that a higher protein intake while losing weight can help to minimise muscle loss while maximising fat loss, particularly when combined with exercise.

This does not mean that you need to follow one of the extreme high-protein, low-carb diets for successful results. The problem with protein when you're trying to lose weight is that it often comes with a lot of undesirable saturated fat. Think of a piece of steak before the fat has been trimmed away. The way to avoid this fat is to go for fish, tofu and tempeh, nuts, eggs and lean meats. Each of your three daily meals should contain 20–25 per cent high-quality protein.

Pasta and grains do contain some protein, but you generally need to supplement this with another source such as seafood on your pasta or nut butter on your toast. We often have a smoothie for breakfast with fruit, yoghurt and flaxseed oil; we include a couple of tablespoonfuls of organic seeds and nuts for protein.

Finally on this subject, the official US nutritional guidelines have just changed to incorporate a wider recommended band of each macronutrient than they did previously. This reflects the fact that we now know there is no one correct ratio for eating. The bottom line is perhaps not to think too much about the ratios. You can choose to eat more protein and fewer carbs — this may suit you if you are less active — but don't cut out the carbs completely, and find quality sources from each group. It's all about balance and discovering what is the best, most enjoyable way of eating for you.

STRATEGY 18 BALANCE YOUR PLATE

Learn to balance your nutritional intake by choosing the right mix of smart carbs, good fats and lean protein. A correctly balanced meal will make you feel full for up to six hours during the day!

Be careful with coffee, alcohol and spicy foods

Some foods actually elevate your metabolic rate more than others; coffee and spicy foods are among these. There's mixed research on the other health benefits of coffee, but the most recent consensus is that the positives seem to outweigh the risks, provided that we drink it in moderation and in a low-fat form.

From a weight-control perspective, the latter is very important. An ordinary cup of black coffee contains virtually no calories, but some of the large-format Starbucks concoctions can contain more than 500! The whipped cream alone in these can add 130 calories, not to mention the array of flavoured syrups on offer. Skip the extras and if you like your coffee white, choose non-fat or low-fat milk.

There is one further note of caution here for those who are particularly sensitive to the effects of caffeine and other stimulant drinks: you don't want to mess with your sleep cycles. We produce some of the main hormones responsible for the regeneration of cell tissues at fixed times during our normal night's sleep. If we go to bed two hours later than usual, we can miss out on our production of these for the day. Over the long term this interferes with our health in all sorts of ways, including our ability to burn calories efficiently. Studies also show that when we're tired we tend to eat more during the day.

If you're having trouble sleeping, you may want to cut coffee out of your diet, or restrict yourself to one cup earlier in the morning. Be careful what you choose as a substitute, though. Many hot chocolates contain more than 300 calories!

Some of the antioxidants in green tea are believed to enhance the effect of caffeine in thermogenisis, but if you're a stress cadet the same rules as for coffee apply; low-caffeine herbal teas are probably a safer, healthier bet for you.

There is evidence that spicy foods, especially those containing chilli, also have a higher than normal thermogenic effect; you should apply the same cautions as for hot drinks. A lot of spicy fast food also has a high fat content — look for low-calorie options.

And with all fast food, don't get taken in by the 'supersize' scam. The major costs in the fast food industry are rent, equipment and wages. The added cost in food that's required to supersize your order is often just a few cents, but can be very expensive to your health. Supersizing is a very, very bad deal.

Alcohol also has few, if any, redeeming features from a weight-loss point of view. Gram for gram it is almost as energy-rich as fat. There are around 100–200 calories in a serving of wine or beer, depending on the size of the glass and the alcohol content. This can quickly add up during a night of socialising. Cocktails typically contain 100–300 calories, but some can have more calories than a Big Mac. And of course a few drinks make you more likely to say yes to a huge, calorie-laden dessert!

The same rules apply to the dietary side of alcohol as to the other health aspects. Limit yourself to 1–2 drinks a day, preferably in the form of wine or a similar lower calorie choice.

STRATEGY 19 CONSUME COFFEE, FAST FOOD AND ALCOHOL WISELY AND IN MODERATION

Modern research has shown that some of the traditional dietary 'sins' may actually contain elements that are beneficial to our health. Part of this, no doubt, comes from the pleasurable psychosocial process of indulging in them. We don't have to become abstinent to maintain a healthy weight, just learn to moderate our vices.

Summary

There are quite a few steps here, but if you take them one at a time none of this is particularly hard to achieve. It's as simple as switching from potato chips to carrots one week, then from full-cream milk to low-fat the next. See our quick summary list in Appendix 1 for help with this. Gradually making small improvements can lead to a massive change in the way you live your life — and in your health. Very soon, you will look back and wonder how you ever ate any differently.

jackie **|** I try to keep it really simple for patients who are trying to lose weight. Three things will kick start most people into the success that drives a continuation of effort:

1. Eat half of your normal-sized evening meal; the other half often makes a great lunch the next day.

2. Have good protein with every meal: it fills you up and maintains your energy levels for longer.

3. Really understand and eat low-GI carbohydrates. Eating these at each meal along with protein is the key to satiation. You need far fewer "snacks".❜

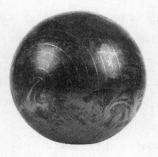

4 | free the mind, the body will follow

Preserve yourself

A few years ago an elderly undertaker was being interviewed on talkback radio. Asked about changes in the profession during his lifetime, he explained that a lot of the pressure had eased in the years after World War 2; as our daily intake of preservatives and pesticides increased, undertakers didn't need to attend to the departed with anything like the urgency required early in his career.

It's no surprise that we don't go off as fast. Our food is crammed full of additives and preservatives, intended to keep it fresh throughout the lengthy journey from 'farm' to dinner table, which has come about as a result of our industrialised agricultural system. Each individual in the developed world consumes 1.3 kg of non-traditional additives and preservatives per year. Our food is further coated with residues of pesticides, herbicides and fungicides meant to kill living things, and each of us ingests about 1 kg of them every year as well. The traditional preservatives like salt, sugar and citric acid that are widely used in our food are not included in these figures, but have their own health implications.

There is a staggering array of these compounds, with conflicting claims about their health effects and safety. Many of them are known carcinogens, hormone disrupters and neurotoxins, and there is virtually no published information on the effects they have when combined, which is how these compounds are consumed. We do know that combinations of pharmaceuticals and drugs like nicotine, caffeine and alcohol have widely varying effects because of the interactions between one drug and others in the human body. But we have no idea what is happening in people when they are exposed to cocktails of synthetic compounds. What's more, we will probably never know because the mixtures are too complicated to allow a sensible research protocol, and the chemicals so universal that it would be hard to prevent an experimental group being exposed while conducting the research. However, there are some facts that cannot be disputed.

Firstly, the number of cancer deaths has dramatically increased. *Environmental and Occupational Causes of Cancer; A Review of Recent Scientific Literature* by Richard Clapp, Genevieve Howe and Molly Jacobs Lefebre, published in 2005, states that between 1950 and 2001 the incidence rate for all types of cancer increased by 85 per cent, using age-adjusted data — which means that more people are getting cancer because they're exposed to more cancer-causing agents, rather than because they're living longer. Fifty per cent of all men and 40 per cent of all women in the US will now hear the words 'You've got cancer' at some point in their lives.

The next thing that is an absolute certainty is that this is not just due to smoking. The growing burden of cancer in children provides some of the most convincing evidence of the role of environmental exposure. Children do not smoke, drink alcohol or hold stressful jobs. In proportion to their bodyweight, however, they drink two and a half times more water, eat three to four times more food, and breathe twice as much air as adults. In addition, their developing bodies may well be affected by parental exposures prior to conception, exposures while growing in the uterus, and the contents of breast milk.

Finally, we know that some people respond to certain compounds, or combinations, far more than others. For example, while it is clear that lung cancer is a leading cause of cancer deaths worldwide, not every smoker will die of it. Similarly, there has been a massive increase in the incidence of asthma among children for reasons that are not completely clear, but there are still some children who do not get the condition — despite being exposed to the same environmental factors. Our contemporary lives in industrial societies have condemned some people to suffer enormously and in many ways this burden has been placed on them unnecessarily. If we had to use chemicals to produce enough food to feed everyone, then the suffering of some might be justified but, as we will see, this is not the case.

As you read through the next few pages you might feel overwhelmed by the enormity of the problem. But the solutions are readily available to almost all of us and we believe everyone who *can* take action, must.

What's been happening down on the farm?

In 1900 in America, 37 out of 100 people worked on farms, but by 1990 the number had dropped to two per cent. There were three main reasons for this massive shift. The first was the availability of cheap oil to power the new mechanised irrigation systems and farm machinery, provide the basis for synthetic fertilisers and distribute the product across thousands of miles.

The second cause was an ongoing obsession with economic efficiency that had begun when Frederick Winslow Taylor introduced 'scientific management' at the Bethlehem Steel Company in 1880, and increased the amount of coal moved per man per day from 16 tons to 59 tons. This was in contrast to the more relaxed small-farm lifestyle developed over centuries in Europe. While the industrial approach may be fine for efficiently delivering cars or guns to market, with food production some essential qualities have ended up being sacrificed in the name of efficiency. We'll look at this in detail a bit later.

The third reason was poor government policy. Under Roosevelt's New Deal policies for recovery from the 1930s Depression, a government loan programme was introduced with the very reasonable aims of keeping farmers in business through times of market downturn and inclement weather, and of creating a national grain reserve to protect people from starvation during hard times. However, Nixon's government changed this from a loan system to one of direct subsidy, which encouraged farmers to produce as much as they possibly could. The end result was a narrow focus on the production of the commodity-grade corn, soy, wheat, rice etc that qualified for the subsidies, at the expense of higher quality, more differentiated crops. This in turn led to mountainous surpluses of these commodities being produced at huge cost to the US taxpayer (government subsidies have amounted to more than a third of many farmers' incomes in recent times).

These forces set in motion centralised industrial agriculture on the scale that we see today, with enormous outputs but tremendous downsides. Since the middle of the 20th century, particularly in the United States, farmers have applied more and more fertiliser, pesticides, herbicides (against weeds) and fungicides (against rotting in storage) to their land and crops, in order to produce yields that would have been beyond the wildest dreams of previous generations.

At first, this achievement seemed like a miracle and proof of man's mastery of the environment via science. But increasingly we are realising that this style of farming is adding to the polluting effects of industrial processing and distribution, and we are seeing the terrible effects those chemicals are having on both people and the environment.

It is also affecting our ability to farm. Industrial agriculture is a major cause of water shortages, topsoil erosion and land being rendered infertile through salinisation. It ignores natural checks and balances, produces massive amounts of waste, depletes fish stocks and other wild food sources, poisons ecosystems and destroys natural habitats. It is a major contributor to greenhouse gas production. The problem is accelerating thanks to population growth and will only get worse as the Third World aspires to First World consumer status. The UN's Millennium Report states that if we do not address these problems very quickly, our present course will have the contrary effect to that which was intended, and by 2050 we will simply not have enough to feed the world.

It is essential to let our decision-makers at every level — in government, industry and agriculture — know exactly what we think and what we want them to do. But we must act now. We, as consumers, can alter these patterns with the one easy recourse we have: our wallets.

How did we get it so wrong?

How did we get so out of sync?

We've mentioned the three big forces that combined in the post-war years to create the industrial agriculture monster, but that is only part of the story. Up until the mid-20th century, farmers grew a range of crops, grazed different animals and maintained soil balances by rotating crops from field to field on a yearly basis. It was a closed system, where the farm animals ate grass and then fertilised the soil and, in the case of pigs, disposed of waste, which was then turned into compost. In this way, the natural fertility of the soil was maintained. Without crop rotation, the soil does not recover and loses its organic content of natural humus, forcing the farmer to use more and more fertiliser to achieve the same output.

Mixed farming ended in much of the world with World War Two and the introduction of industrial mono-crop farming. Big food companies started to contract farmers to produce a single crop, which created business and farm efficiencies — at least in the short term. Developments in the science of farming meant that farmers could dramatically boost production through the use of fertiliser, pesticides, herbicides and fungicides. By focusing on one or two crops, farmers could create efficiencies in equipment and storage, essentially becoming more industrial and for the first time emerging from their traditional hard-working lifestyle. Michael Pollan notes in his book *The Omnivore's Dilemma* (our number one reading recommendation for further understanding in this area) that American farmers in the post-war era were, for the first time in history, able to take winter holidays in Florida — *if* they could afford it.

The big food companies created massive distribution networks, dependent, of course, on oil for distributing those crops to supermarkets across the country and around the world. This process created business efficiencies in the short term, but in the long term farmers became imprisoned by the system. Their produce became commodities sold on distant trading floors and the distinctive local fruit and vegetables that had developed to suit particular climates and particular soils lost value and were abandoned. More than 2000 vegetable varieties were lost between 1975 and 1995. Over-production of basic foodstuffs in some markets also led to a fall in prices.

The case of the Idaho potato farmers is a classic example. It has been replicated in one form or another all over the industrialised world and for every popular type of fruit or vegetable, from apples to zucchini. Idaho potato farmers shifted to a uniform size, shape and texture for the fast food industry; in particular, they bred a potato that was perfect for making the French fries ubiquitous in American fast food restaurants. When you are selling to a limited number of customers you are in a very vulnerable position, and very quickly the fast food companies effectively owned the potato growers. They gave exact specifications about the potatoes: the size, shape, texture, starch levels and the exact length of storage times. This allowed the fast food companies to increase their efficiencies because they only had to deal with one type of potato. But such tight mono-cropping tends to make plants vulnerable to pests and diseases, because the pests learn where the crops are and what their weaknesses are. So the farmers had to apply more and more 'inputs' to the crops, i.e. dousing them with chemicals.

This downward spiral resulted in ever-growing expenses and lower net returns to farmers, which in turn led to consolidation of farms and fewer and fewer farmers. This is not just a historical phenomenon and is not restricted to the US. The number of fruit and vegetable growers in New Zealand declined from 7000 to 2000 in the five years from 2001–2006.

Would you like oil with that?

The quantities of fertiliser that we are talking about are massive. In 1914, New Zealand was a farming country and already an exporter of meat and dairy products to England. In that year we applied 1200 tonnes of nitrogen fertiliser nationwide. By 1971 this had increased to around 2.2 million tonnes, roughly a two thousand-fold increase. By 1996 the figure had leapt to 3.1 million tonnes and this solid fertiliser was supplemented by 2.6 million litres of concentrated liquid fertiliser. So approximately 40 per cent more fertiliser was applied in 1996 than in 1971, yet over the same period there was a significant decline in some farming sectors due to the removal of subsidies. In round figures, New Zealand is applying about one tonne of fertiliser per year for each person living here! Even crazier, almost all of this fertiliser is of fossil fuel origin, from either oil or natural gas, and all is imported. Quite simply, we are using oil to import fertiliser made from oil and then using oil to export foodstuffs. Our customers are eating oil!

Fertilisers cause environmental problems at every level, but mostly because we overuse them. There is a highly developed science behind fertiliser application, but farmers are human beings like the rest of us, and businesspeople as well. The temptation to apply just a bit more — even though it's expensive — to guarantee a good crop is sometimes just too great.

One of the effects of overuse is the creation of dead zones. Fertiliser running into the Mississippi River has created one such zone in the Gulf of Mexico that is the size of New Jersey. It has caused massive fish deaths and economic damage in surrounding areas. Similar situations exist in the Baltic Sea, the Black Sea and many other bodies of water, including some of our own lakes and shorelines in New Zealand.

We talk in Chapter 8 of the colossal volcanic eruptions that formed Lake Taupo in the centre of the North Island around 2000 years ago. Today this vast lake also has dead zones, with high levels of some pollutants, especially nitrates, from agricultural run-off. Steps are being taken to limit fertiliser application in the lake's catchments but it is expected that it will take as long as 80 years to see any difference. We take off our hats to the decision-makers involved in that piece of foward thinking and hope their leadership is remembered in 80 years' time.

If enormous bodies of water in remote countries like New Zealand have measurable levels of agricultural pollutants, there are not likely to be many places on Earth — including the Arctic and Antarctica — which are free of them. The Arctic has been affected because of a system known as global distillation. Essentially, the farmer who is applying agrichemicals in Central America is unintentionally helping to poison Inuit babies in northern Canada. Some of the spray is elevated into the atmosphere and moves north with the prevailing winds until the colder conditions drive it down to surface level and it gets into the food chain. It's eaten by zooplankton, which is essential food for fish, and then by progressively larger creatures until it winds up in one of the mammals traditionally hunted by Inuit.

Just like global warming, this is a harsh lesson that has unfolded during our lifetimes. We used to think that environmental damage happened locally: near the oil spill or the factory belching smoke, or alongside the forest that was being chopped down, but now it is obvious that our activities are having a truly global impact. The internationally renowned primatologist Dr Jane Goodall states in her book *Harvest for Hope: A Guide to Mindful Eating* that farm chemicals currently kill up to 67 million birds a year in the United States. She also quotes studies on the dramatic effects of farm chemicals on the incidence of cancer, Parkinson's disease, miscarriages and birth defects, and on children's health and mental development.

An organic revolution

What can we possibly do when we are faced with such dire side effects from industrial farming? Fortunately, the answer is simple — and has been tested in farm-scale trials and in one entire country for over a decade. It is to move our agricultural activities over to organic production. Many people will be thinking that organic farming is the stuff of hippies and communes, or at best a boutique option that only the wealthiest can afford. Some will be thinking that it is less productive and we will not be able to feed the world. But this is not the case.

Sometimes the truth is scary

There are stages in our acceptance of a new truth. Initially we dismiss it out of hand, make disparaging jokes about it and link it with mad conspiracy theories. Then, slowly, we start to accept it. Sound familiar? We've seen this occur with smoking and health; CFCs and the ozone layer; greenhouse gases and climate change. Now it is happening with organic farming.

The country we mentioned is Cuba. With a population of more than 11 million people, it was forced to transform its agricultural sector from one that was based on Soviet industrial agriculture, with massive inputs of oil-based fertiliser, insecticide, herbicide and fungicide, into one based on organic techniques with far fewer inputs of fuel. This change was forced on Cuba almost overnight by the collapse of the Soviet Union. From being a large sugar-producing country subsidised with inputs of oil, money, fertiliser and agrichemicals from the Soviet empire, it became one that had to provide for its own diverse requirements. There were lean years in the early 1990s while the new systems were put in place, but for over a decade the new organic sector has been more productive and produced more nutritious food in a far greater variety than was available before.

And if you don't trust Fidel (although the Cuban results have been widely monitored by reputable sources), the home of centralised industrial agriculture is also feeling the winds of change. In the past decade, organic food sales in the United States have increased tenfold; if this rate of growth continues, most of the food sold in the US by 2020 will be organic. In *Harvest for Hope*, Dr Goodall notes that sales of organic produce grew from US$1 billion to US$11 billion in the 12 years from 1990. In 1997, 485,000 hectares of land were devoted to organic farming; by 2001 that had doubled to 930,800 hectares. Perhaps even more interestingly, she notes that the top 25 per cent of farmers following sustainable organic practices now have higher yields than the nation's industrial farms. As in Cuba, the produce is better for the consumer, tastier and better for the environment.

Politically, one of the interesting things about reading the early literature from the 1940s on organic farming is that the people involved could not have been more conservative; they included engineers, orchardists and scientists. In 1947, when a petition regarding the need to maintain the quality of soil humus was forwarded to the New Zealand Parliament, it was supported by the local branch of the British Medical Association. These people were not 'mad greenies' as we sometimes hear modern-day organic devotees called. That reactionary attitude has probably stemmed from two things: firstly, the politics of the right shifting away from any serious conservative base towards its large corporate suitors, and secondly, people being lulled into a false sense of security by the large harvest that's been delivered to our supermarkets by cheap oil.

We now need to start looking into the unfolding market for organics a bit more thoroughly.

Tastier and healthier

Organic food tastes better and it is more nutritious. Neither claim should come as any surprise. Organic growers and the consumers of their produce have known this all along, but we now have evidence to back them up. Industrially produced fruit and vegetables are bred for consistent size, shape and colour rather than flavour. Commercial imperatives such as storage time take precedence over taste, so it's small wonder that we wind up with bland, flavourless produce. Many organic growers are trying to salvage tasty heritage varieties that we may remember from our childhoods.

In respect of our health, Michael Pollan quotes recent University of California studies showing organic food to have significantly higher levels of vitamins and other micronutrients such as polyphenols. The latter are a group of plant substances recently discovered to be crucial in preventing cancers and in optimising our nutrition. And of course, by eating organic we avoid the risk of exposing ourselves to the insecticides, fungicides, hormones, antibiotics and other chemicals present in industrially grown meat and produce, more and more of which are being found to have terrible effects on human biology.

About now, you need to banish thoughts of the organic shops of old, with their wizened old vegetables, dusty shelves and bins of mung beans. The organic food industry has evolved and has got much better at fulfilling customers' expectations. Take our local shop, Harvest Wholefoods in Grey Lynn, Auckland, which has expanded over the years and is now a sleek, organised store with an excellent selection of organic fruit and vegetables. Its heart is still the same, but it has really lifted its game as a retailer and the long checkout queues will quickly show you just how mainstream the organic movement has become. Working at our office in Southern California is paradise for us in terms of food shopping, with organic supermarkets, co-ops and farmers' markets everywhere — although we are cautioned by Michael Pollan's exposé of shallow versus deep organics in the US (more on this below).

Organics online

We were sharing some of our ideas with our younger staff members and were surprised by how many had grown up without ever having a vege garden at home; as a result, they have no real idea about which fruit and vegetables are harvested in each of the seasons. One of them said: 'If the fruit and veges are cheap, they must be in season.' Her logic is right, but these days it's getting easier to be sure.

In lots of cities and towns, small farmers and gardeners are joining together to offer organic vege deliveries. You simply pay your $20 or $40 and every week a box of fruit and vegetables gets delivered to your door. What's exciting is that you never know what you're going to receive, because you only get what's in season, ripe and ready to eat.

We have friends in Christchurch who order organic beef online from a farm on the outskirts of the city and it is delivered to their door once a week. They can also add organic poultry, eggs and lamb to their online requests.

Farmers' markets are also enjoying a resurgence in popularity and some have tight controls about the rules of entry. Only organic produce grown locally can be sold at many of them.

Increasingly, there are initiatives like these everywhere. A great way to influence the future is to search online for the organic providers in your neighbourhood and shop there. Then, ring your local supermarket owner to say you'll be back when they start stocking more organic products.

No pain, no gain?

The price of organic food has dropped, although there is still a differential. However, as people we know have found, if you're cutting out junk food then you will have more cash in your budget! Besides, the grocery store price does not reflect how much we pay for our damaged health and weakened immune systems. Yes, organic food does cost a little more, but can you put a price on the well-being of your family?

There's also the argument that with the billions of dollars that go into subsidising the food industry in the United States and elsewhere, consumers in those countries are actually paying a huge amount more for that food through their taxes than just the price on the shelf.

And it's almost impossible to measure how much we spend trying to clean up and cope with environmental damage caused by chemical intensive farming. Goodall notes that the Rodale Institute calculated that America could comply with the Kyoto Treaty's demand for a reduction in greenhouse gases, simply by making a full switch to organic farming. Centralised industrial agriculture uses much more fossil fuel than organic production.

There is a growing awareness of the link between sustainability and continued economic prosperity. People are realising that we can no longer continue in the way that we have been, sucking the resources out of the earth without thinking about the effect, and then dousing it with chemicals to increase the return.

If you can't beat 'em, buy 'em

The massive growth of the organic sector has brought its own problems. We need to take a closer look at how the unfolding market for organic produce is developing. In an interview published on the outstanding website *www.rachel. org* recently, veteran commentator and activist Ronnie Cummins noted that in the United States, about ten cents in every food dollar is spent on organic food — and that is growing dramatically. Naturally enough, large corporations have seen this trend and are starting to take over the organic sector and degrade the organic standards.

'Right now,' Cummins told *rachel.org*, 'forty per cent of organic milk is coming from Horizon Organic and Aurora Organic, producers who are both practising intensive confinement of farm animals, allowing them no access to pasture. They're also regularly importing calves from industrial farms and simply calling them organic. These heifers have been weaned on antibiotics and fed slaughterhouse waste and GMO grains ... This is not helping thousands of humane family-scale farmers make the transition to organic. Instead, they are changing the rules and allowing industrial agriculture to call it organic.'

As part of the takeover of the industry, there is the corporate takeover of organic food brands. This is a major trend, with many producers not printing the names of their parent corporation on the label, perhaps because they know that those corporations have such a terrible reputation with organic consumers; if we knew, we would be unlikely to want to buy their products. Also, they often do not list the country of origin on the labels, so organic consumers buy their products while remaining in the dark about where and by whom they were produced.

Deep versus shallow

Essentially, there is a growing distinction between what you might call 'deep' organic and 'shallow' organic. Both Pollan and Goodall have written about the tenets of deep organic farming as opposed to its shallow cousin. In deep organics, farmers are committed to biodiversity — raising different types of plants and animals that are rotated around the fields to enrich the soil and help prevent disease and pest outbreaks.

Resources such as water, soil and air are respected and replenished so that the farmers sustain the ecosystem and cause no harm to future generations. The waste within the farm ecosystem doesn't contaminate the bordering land, air or waterways. Agrichemicals are not used unless absolutely necessary, and then only with great caution and the minimum application possible. Animals are treated humanely and are well cared for. They are permitted to carry out their natural behaviour such as grazing, rooting or pecking, and are fed a natural diet appropriate for their species. Farmers are properly compensated, and workers are treated fairly and paid competitive wages and benefits, operating in a safe environment and offered healthy living conditions and food. The farm contributes to the local food distribution, minimising cost, handling, packaging and pollution caused by long-distance transportation.

On the other hand, shallow organic, according to Goodall, 'still participates in an infrastructure that favours mass production, excessive packaging and shipping food thousands of miles to the grocery store. Shallow organic still needs lots of oil and short-term fixes. In the end, shallow organic's success is measured by profit, not sustainability.'

Pollan points out that the industrial establishment has lobbied the USDA to weaken its organic standards, and that big organic farms now engage in practices like mono-cropping, and over-tilling the soil to kill weeds; in the process, they are sterilising natural soil humus and removing its nutritional qualities.

Is food really organic if it's shipped in cool storage halfway across the world to a distribution centre, trucked to the store and then wrapped up in plastic? Some would argue that buying organic produce that's been brought to your country on a cargo ship isn't exactly good for the environment. Such food is not truly organic or sustainable, they suggest. Instead, it's simply plugging organics into our pre-existing expectations of what food we should be able to eat — and when. The idea that you can eat aubergines or asparagus in winter is what caused many of the problems in the first place.

Personally, we take a sensible approach. In the first instance, we buy local whenever we can. We try to buy products that fit into the 'deep organic' mould. By doing this you will ease the transport burden on the environment, reduce the use of sprays and eat better.

If you can't buy local organic, you're still ahead. There's no doubt that it's better not to use so many chemicals. And the New Zealand Ministry for the Environment has calculated that in terms of your global footprint — a measure of how much effect a person has on the world's environment — it's better to eat organic food, wherever it's from. Of course, in terms of the benefit to your own health you're far and away better off.

Again, it's a game of inches. We can't do everything. If you simply cannot get something locally, or if the only available organic product is imported, it is still generally better to eat organic than non-organic.

Read the label

All of this simply underscores the need to have clear food labelling and to get to know your food retailer. What you can do is demand better labelling on the one hand and on the other, only buy products that are adequately labelled. There are all sorts of discussions around what is —and is not — organic, and there are all sorts of standards. Get informed, find the relevant information sources through the web and make your own decisions about the value of the different certifying bodies. You will find some very good information in organic outlets and health food stores as well. Ultimately, consumer demand and information technology will make a big contribution in this area. Already in Denmark you can scan a barcode at a terminal and get a range of information that's as detailed as the farm of origin, its farming practices and its philosophies.

There are other good things happening, too. In large part because of consumer pressure, the broader farm industry is becoming more health-oriented. In New Zealand there has been a huge movement away from using insecticides in fruit orchards, for example. All kiwifruit now grown in this country is produced to very green standards. The industry uses minimal amounts of agricultural spray, about ten per cent of what was used in the early 1990s. It's the same with apples and most other New Zealand fruit. There were fears about trade barriers being put up in Europe against the importation of New Zealand apples and kiwifruit, so there have been programmes to dramatically reduce the amount of spraying.

Eat less meat

Meat production has increased by 500 per cent since 1950. Consumption increased worldwide to a staggering 276 million tons in 2006. How has the centralised agricultural industry achieved that kind of growth? Well, for a start they haven't done it in fields. Most animals today in the United States are reared on industrial factory farms where the animals are crowded into enclosures and fed industrial corn and hormones rather than grass. This causes problems in their digestive systems and, because of the overcrowding, leaves them susceptible to getting sick. To prevent this they are given antibiotics. The World Watch Institute (which has an information-rich website, *www.worldwatch.org*) has estimated that around 70 per cent of all antibiotics used in the United States are given to pigs, chicken and cows to try to make up for the dirty, cramped conditions that these animals are subjected to on factory farms. World Watch reported that a 2002 study found that 37 per cent of chickens sampled in major grocery stores were contaminated with antibiotic-resistant pathogens.

Aside from the effects on your health from eating these pathogens, factory farming has a calamitous impact on the environment. It produces huge concentrations of manure that has to go somewhere; on a traditional farm, manure is recycled as fertiliser, but on a feedlot it's waste. In 2006, factory farms in the United States produced 132,000 mllion tonnes of manure each day, about six times more than humans. There have been some disastrous spills. In 1995, nine and a half million litres of effluent was spilled into the New River, North Carolina, from a pig farm and it killed ten million fish.

The production of meat creates a very large ecological footprint. As with this whole subject, you have to follow the food chain back to see the real effect. To raise animals in this way, they are fed many times their body weight every year, which means a vast acreage of grains, soybeans and corn. The World Health Organisation and the Food and Agriculture Organisation of the

United Nations have estimated that you can feed 22 people for a year from growing one hectare of potatoes and 19 people a hectare with rice. You can feed just one or two people per year growing beef from the product of the same area. The US Department of Agriculture's Economic Research Service has estimated that it takes 16 kg of grain to produce one kg of beef. The vast majority of grains and soybeans in the world are being produced to support the farming industry.

At the same time, huge tracts of rainforests in South America, literally the lungs of our planet, are being destroyed to create fields for growing soy feed, which is shipped overseas to animal feedlots and battery farms. Choosing industrially produced steak or chicken for dinner is in this way directly contributing to global warming.

The industrial farming of feed crops also exposes the soil to erosion and salt build up. It is variously estimated that between one fifth and one third of the planet's prime arable land has been rendered unusable by centralised industrial agricultural practices. Put very simply, the meat side of contemporary agriculture is anything but sustainable, except in organic farms and in countries where animals are still primarily fed on grass, such as New Zealand.

Different animals have different effects. Pig farming tends to be done on feedlots. This creates huge amounts of pollution, in particular large amounts of nitrogen from all of the sewage that they produce. Not only does that result in the poisoning of nearby waterways, but nitrous oxide is also a very powerful greenhouse gas — it has 310 times the effect, molecule for molecule, of carbon dioxide on climate change.

Industrial meat farming uses massive amounts of water. Producing one kg of soybeans or rice requires about 2000 litres of water. It takes approximately 3500 litres to produce one kg of chicken. A single kg of beef uses 100,000 litres.

What goes in must come out. Cattle are responsible for a significant contribution to greenhouse gases through the emission of methane. It is a major greenhouse gas, 21 times more powerful than carbon dioxide as a greenhouse gas on a molecule-for-molecule basis. Because of methane, meat production in the United States is responsible for about a quarter of greenhouse gas creation.

In New Zealand, our cows and sheep are still pasture-fed. As Michael Pollan says, in grass farming the primary energy source is the sun. From that perspective, New Zealand is clean and green. But because it is a farming nation and has a very low population compared with its size, methane from farm animals is our major contribution to global warming. This is something that we as a country are trying to deal with.

We do not believe that people need to become vegetarians or vegans. In our family, for instance, we often eat vegetarian meals, but we eat lean organic steak or lamb once a week, organic free-range chicken once a week and fish from ecologically friendly sources (more on this below) three or four times a week.

We believe that humans are designed to consume small amounts of meat, and on the whole it is healthy for us occasionally to eat lean organic meat that is not contaminated with hormones, antibiotics or other man-made compounds. Having said that, we need to be sensible. As a society we consume far too much meat, which is not good for our health (it contributes to heart disease and other illnesses) and — as we have seen — it has a negative impact on the planet.

Smarter farming

A lot of other changes are now taking place in agriculture. Smart farmers are now planting anti-pollution belts beside the lakes or streams on their land, which include native planting or even crops that thrive on nitrogen. These reduce the amount of fertilisers draining into waterways and polluting the ecosystem. In 2003 the Dairying and Clean Streams Accord was signed by New Zealand regional councils, the Ministry for the Environment, the Ministry of Agriculture and Forestry, and dairy farmers who supply the major dairy processor, Fonterra. It was intended to minimise the effect of dairy farming on water quality. The agreement aimed to have 100 per cent of farms effectively managing nutrient run-off by 2007 and to have them dealing with effluent discharges immediately.

This initiative was presented as 'an industry-backed accord to improve the environmental performance of dairy farming', with the intention that it would 'send a strong message to the public and to domestic and international consumers, that environmental management is an integral and important component of the dairy industry.'

The big GM

If consumers want to move to organic produce and are shopping accordingly, many in the corporate world of agribusiness are placing their bets in another direction: genetic engineering. In terms of short-term profits they may be right; investors may be dazzled by the PR spin and promised future returns, and buy their shares at inflated prices. Farmers, food consumers or serious financial analysts are likely to be less impressed; spectacular results have been notably absent and the concerns about potential health or environmental effects remain unresolved.

Few areas of the agriculture business have attracted such a variety of responses, ranging from a substantial yawn, initially, in the US, through to very strong resistance in countries as far apart as Germany and India. New Zealand still does not allow imports of genetically modified grain for human consumption, but is in the process of considering an application for GM corn to be grown for animal feed.

We need to go back to basics to try to assess this technology for ourselves. In 1973, American scientists Stanley Cohen of Stanford University and Herbert Boyer of the University of California announced that they had successfully recombined the DNA from two different organisms. In 1974, Paul Berg, an American biologist, called for a moratorium on GM research in areas which might have serious effects on people's health. Although widely supported, his call didn't stop research marching on. It gained particular support from the agribusiness giants, who saw enormous potential after the US Supreme Court ruled that it was possible to patent novel life forms. This opened the possibility of entering the market with new products and plant varieties that would then need new herbicides, in addition to those already being manufactured by the agri-giants.

Like those involved in the nuclear industry, the scientists in this activity are intensely focused on their narrow endeavours. They, or their PR departments, insist that they are operating with a level of precision that in reality is not possible, and they claim that their work is without risk when they cannot possibly know this to be true.

A few simple observations can be made. There has been no attempt to build up peer-reviewed literature on the safety of genetically modified organisms (GMOs). This is the normal way that scientific advances are reported and while some sectors, like the pharmaceutical industry, are criticised for selectively releasing data from safety studies, they are at least taking part in them.

There are several distinct potential hazards associated with GMOs that *are* reported in scientific literature (please excuse the technical language):

- Synthetic genes and gene products which are new to evolution could be toxic to humans and other animals or provoke serious immune reactions.

- The uncontrollable, imprecise process involved in making GMOs can generate unintended toxic and immunogenic products, exacerbated by the instability of the transgenic lines.

- Naturally occuring viruses that cause disease could be activated by the transgenic process.

- The synthetic genes in GMOs, including copies of genes from bacteria and viruses that cause disease as well as antibiotic resistance genes, may be transferred to other species via pollen, or by direct integration into other genomes in horizontal gene transfer.

- Under natural conditions, disease-causing viruses and bacteria are created by horizontal gene transfer and recombination. Genetic modification mimics this process, and might be expected to greatly enhance the creation of disease-causing agents.

- GM DNA is designed to invade genomes, and insertion into the genomes of animals, including human beings, results in insertion mutagenesis, some of which may trigger cancer.

- Herbicide-tolerant GM crops accumulate herbicide and herbicide residues that could be highly toxic to humans and animals as well as plants.

Getting to the bottom of each of these issues is a job for highly trained specialists, and debate should be happening in a public forum without the pressure of shareholders wanting an immediate financial return on their investments.

Overall, the risk profile for genetic engineering appears to be much like that for the nuclear industry, although the use of living things introduces an element of further unpredictability. The probability of a major health or environmental issue arising from GMOs may be low, but the consequences if one did occur could be huge, potentially even larger than from a major nuclear accident.

Put simply, there is no way of containing a GMO that has been released into the environment. An even simpler way of measuring risk is to ask whether those involved have insurance coverage for every, or any, eventuality. The fact is that they generally do not, because the insurers cannot assess the risks.

Reports already published suggest that genetically modified corn has crossed with wild varieties in Mexico and that herbicide-resistance qualities introduced as a GMO are appearing in wild strains of weed species. Monsanto, a major producer of GM seeds, has even sued farmers whose crops have been contaminated by their GMO variety for patent infringement!

From the nascent research we have seen on the health effects of GMO food, there is no way we would feed it to our family — or to anyone. When the stakes are so high we have to demand a moratorium on further use of GMOs in the field until some serious environmental impact assessment work is carried out.

STRATEGY 20 EAT FOR THE PLANET

Organics are not just for hippies. Green is the new black. It's cool. Hollywood is on board and the issues around eating for the planet are making strange bedfellows of liberal conservationists and conservative business people who are rethinking the sustainability of the 'bigger is better' logic. The truth can't be denied.

There are simple actions you can take immediately. Buy organic food produced locally. Eat less meat. Steer well clear

of anything that's been genetically modified. And enjoy the subsequent improvements to your well-being, as well as your gift to the planet.

And there's one more thing: don't forget that letter or phone call to your local supermarket. Your opinion might just be the one that tips the scales.

If something seems fishy, it probably is . . .

phillip **'** In the late 1960s, my schoolmate Philip Gould and I would occasionally play hookey and take our dinghy from Meola Creek near his house, to a fishing spot on the other side of Auckland's Waitemata Harbour. We were able to catch a seemingly endless haul of fish there, and we soon found there was a ready market for this as pet food through our neighbourhood grocery store.

These fishing trips were so successful that we expanded our operation, with the addition of a friend's net. We'd block off part of Meola Creek for a few hours and haul in as much as 20 pounds of sprats. We were on our way to making a tidy sum, when the creek ran out of fish. We tried again from time to time over the next year, but the numbers of fish never increased and we eventually moved on to other things. In my adult years I've looked back in shame, wondering how long it took the schools of fish in that creek to recover.

Every time I have told this story, all over the world, I have found someone my age or older who has a variation — from their own childhood, in their own lake, river or patch of sea. In *Under the Bridge and Over the Moon*, New Zealand writer Kevin Ireland tells his story of maritime plunder in the 1940s. He and a school friend had a competition about the relative merits of fishing just off the beaches closest to their respective homes. Ireland won the bet in grand style when the two boys caught 84 snapper in one session off Takapuna Beach; they barely had sufficient freeboard to row their boat ashore without sinking and losing the lot. **'**

But even repeating these childhood antics a million times all over the planet would make only a tiny contribution to the conclusion reached by a scientific team at the end of 2006: that we are likely to have used all of the seafood in the world's oceans by 2048. A team of 14 ecologists and economists drew this stunning conclusion based on the evidence that they can find on the state of the world's fisheries up until 2003.

The *Washington Post*, which reported this study, said the authors have come in for criticism from other fisheries specialists, who suggest that quotas and other conservation measures introduced in the USA and New Zealand, among other countries, will save the day.

This is a familiar situation. One group of scientists paints an alarming picture; others say they are being too pessimistic. We have seen the same scenario played out on everything from ozone holes to climate change. The challenge for each of us is to gauge the most probable outcome when we are presented with competing theories: one which predicts disaster and requires immediate action; another which concludes there is no problem at all, thereby allowing us to remain comfortably complacent.

As individuals, how can we possibly make a judgement about the merits of the arguments put before us? In most cases you need years of specialist training before you can make sense of the issues and the numbers involved. You could retrain as a fisheries scientist and might then be able to answer questions about the future of seafood in a few decades' time; but you would still not be equipped to pass any more than layman's comment on climate change or topsoil depletion. There has to be an easier way and fortunately there is: common sense.

In the fisheries example, ask yourself whether the alarmist proposition is remotely plausible, based on your own experience or that of people you have met. The fishermen Phillip has met around the world share his experience of having known small local fisheries that collapsed, sometimes in part because of their contributions.

Next, ask yourself if this could possibly happen on a larger scale. On the internet, for instance, you will find examples of species of animals and birds being wiped out, even when there were far fewer people. Google 'great auk' and you will read about the demise of a large flightless bird known as the northern hemisphere penguin. Unusually, there is an actual date recorded for its final extinction — 3 July, 1844 — when the last known living pair and one egg were captured in Iceland.

Great auks were caught for food and oil, and their feathers used for down bedding in Victorian England. Look up moa or New Zealand eagle and you will find other magnificent birds, including the largest eagle of all time, which became extinct within a few hundred years of humans arriving in their world. If these examples spark your interest, then read some of the books written by the 2007 Australian of the Year, Tim Flannery, for a fascinating history of man's trail of destruction (*The Future Eaters* is about Australia, *The Eternal Frontier* looks at North America). Or check out Jared Diamond's *Collapse*, an analysis of societies throughout history that have failed as a result of ecological abuses. This history is not something to feel guilty about, as it happened generations before our time, but these books provide cautionary examples of what humans can do to the world around them.

So, as regards our fish, we now have a plausible story that passes the 'experience' test of historical examples of species being exterminated. But could seafood supplies really plummet as far as the scientists predict? Closer reading of the *Washington Post* article provided this observation: 'This phenomenon is visible in Maryland's Chesapeake Bay, where the collapse of the oyster fishery has reverberated across the ecosystem. In 1880, there were enough oysters to filter all the water in the bay in three days; by 1988 it took more than a year for the remaining oysters to accomplish the same task.' We have to assume that the few remaining oysters cannot do the job, and without a natural, living filter the water itself is dying out or dead. Barren seas seem plausible to us.

One final test can be applied, and this is a variation of the 'precautionary principle' which receives a lot of discussion in the environmental literature. Google 'precautionary principle' if you want to be boggled by words, but for our purposes just ask yourself what the two proponents at opposite ends of the spectrum want us to do, and what would be the outcome if we follow their advice and they turn out to have been right or wrong.

The fisheries scientists with their alarming research want us to pressure governments to introduce more stringent controls on fishers everywhere. If we follow their advice — and if they are right — there will be fish in the oceans for our children, but in the meantime the cost of fish will almost certainly go up. If they are wrong, and there never was much cause for great concern, the price of fish will go up in the near future and then decline greatly as the superabundance of fish reasserts itself and we are back to the days described in the fishing exploits of Phillip's childhood, or back even further with Kevin Ireland and fish catches so vast that they had the capacity to sink small boats!

If we apply the same logic to those promoting the status quo, at the other end of the spectrum, we see some interesting results. They presumably want us to carry on consuming fish in the same way as we have for many years, and leave them to get on with catching them and selling them to us so they can make money. If they are right and there is no cause for concern, because things are in hand, then there will be ample stocks of fish for the foreseeable future.

This seems unlikely, as the quantity of fish taken from wild fisheries worldwide peaked a number of years ago, and world population continues to increase and, in countries like India and China, get far wealthier. If they are wrong, however, we get back to the fisheries scientists' grim predictions and face a future with barren oceans and children who will never have fish in their diet or experience the delight of catching a fish in the wild.

It's a fishy business

Common sense aside, there are plenty of statistics available.

During Phillip's time at UCLA in the 1970s, one of his and his roommates' staple meals was boiled Atlantic cod and vegetables. The demise of the cod fishery off the Grand Banks is one of the most spectacular collapses of this type worldwide, and it occurred under the watchful eyes of Canadian fisheries scientists who later admitted to getting their numbers wrong. In their excellent book *The Ethics of What We Eat*, Peter Singer and Jim Mason tell the story of the collapse of this fishery from being the most productive in the world to virtual extinction. The adult cod population deteriorated to the point that in 1992 it was an estimated 1.1 per cent of the total in the early 1960s. Despite the fishery's closure in 1992, it has still not recovered and may never do so.

A world away, at the time our children were born in the 1980s, we were introduced to a delicate, white-fleshed fish called orange roughy. It is caught on ocean ridges far off New Zealand's coast and was called slime fish until those trying to market it intervened. Despite government efforts at fisheries management using a quota-management system they claim is leading the world, current stocks are down to five per cent of the pristine stock of a quarter of a century ago.

In 1995, an official with the Fishery Resources Division of the Food and Agricultural Organisation (FAO) of the UN gave the total world fish production for 1993 as 101.4 million tonnes, with 85.7 million tonnes (84.5 per cent) coming from capture fisheries and 15.7 million tonnes from aquaculture (15.5 per cent). The official noted: 'The world's fisheries have reached an apparent level of stabilisation of total catch, which really represents a considerable degree of over-exploitation, as most stocks are degraded in composition and size structure at this level.'

In 2004, total fish production worldwide was 140.5 million tonnes, 38.6 per cent up on production nine years earlier. This was made up of 95 million tonnes from capture fisheries and 45.5 million tonnes from aquaculture, with 67 per cent of the fish farming taking place on small holdings in China. The capture fishery had actually *increased* by 10.85 per cent in less than a decade, which is both remarkable and scary considering it was starting from a state of over-exploitation at that time. The issue facing us now is immediate, drastic action to curb fishing so that the remaining wild stocks can be preserved.

The increase in aquaculture production between 1995 and 2004 was a massive 29.8 million tonnes — nearly 200 per cent — giving hope that pressure on the natural fisheries might be relieved. Sadly, as the British historian Professor Simon Schama has stated: 'History has a cruel way with optimism.' The reality of much fish and prawn farming bears this out, as we shall see.

Possible solutions

Fish provides the single largest source of protein for much of humanity, but 70 per cent of the world's fisheries are in decline. At a time when increasing numbers of people around the globe can afford to pay for fish, the stocks are just not there. There will be more pressure on fish stocks in the future, yet for at least half a century the industry has not been run in a sustainable manner. There is strong evidence to suggest that the global fishing fleet is two and a half times larger than is needed to catch the sustainable yield from the world's oceans.

Faced with these facts, many organisations have prepared some version of a 'good-fish guide' for consumers. In Britain, the Marine Conservation Society has produced an online version at *www.fishonline.org* and Project Aware — *www.projectaware.org* — is trying to keep up with American and

Australian guidelines. The Monterey Bay aquarium's *Seafood Watch* and Environmental Defence's *Oceans Alive* programmes also monitor and rate stocks in US waters. In New Zealand, the Royal Forest and Bird Protection Society has produced a *Best Fish Guide*, a wallet-sized booklet which codes fisheries according to their sustainability: green for good, orange for fisheries where there are concerns around the management of stocks, and red for those that are poorly managed. In the two years since they started producing this guide, they have yet to classify a fishery as green, while many are on the orange list. We recommend studying your local version of the above guides and, when you are at the fish shop, buying only the least threatened species. Let's be quite clear, though: this alone will not be enough.

The next option with fisheries, as we have seen, is aquaculture, and this needs to be divided into three distinct groups: the low-technology production of herbivorous fish, such as carp, in farm ponds in China and India; the high-tech production of high-value carnivorous species, such as salmon and prawns, for the lucrative export market; and the farming of filter-feeding shellfish like mussels and oysters. The first type produces perhaps 70–80 per cent of the total global yield. This low-tech activity is integrated with the other components of a peasant farm and appears to be sustainable, producing a high-quality protein without the use of antibiotics and without the side effect of vast quantities of waste.

The second type of production looks very impressive in its packaged form in the supermarket or in promotional videos. The truth is somewhat different. To begin with, something like 20 per cent of all the fish caught in the wild are turned into fishmeal, which is then fed to salmon being bred at fish farms. Singer and Mason state in *The Ethics of What We Eat* that it takes three to four tonnes of fishmeal to produce a tonne of salmon. The problem with this, they point out, is that it encourages fishermen to take millions of tonnes of small fish that would otherwise provide food for wild fish and, directly or indirectly, feed coastal people in developing countries. Alternative feed sources for salmon are often dubious, such as chicken waste.

Other problems inherent in aquaculture include the use of antibiotics because of the super-crowded conditions in which the fish are kept and, as with other factory farms, there are often issues around waste as huge amounts of uneaten food and salmon effluent enter waterways.

One more problem with fish farming of this nature is that some of the fish chosen to be feedstock for the fishmeal factory are carnivores. This has the effect of increasing the concentration of dioxins, PCBs and other contaminants accumulated in environment because we have added another carnivore to the top of the food chain. Independent tests on the farmed product have borne this out.

Prawn and shrimp farming is also a problem. As with salmon farming, the logic has been well intended, because wild shrimp and prawn fishing is particularly unsustainable. The majority of the shrimp available — about 75 per cent — is caught wild by trawlers using giant conical nets over estuaries, bays and continental shelves, according to Dave Tilford from The Center for the New American Dream, an organisation that encourages Americans to 'consume responsibly to protect the environment'. Tilford says: 'Trawlers scour the seabed in a manner likened to forest clear-cutting, destroying habitat and scooping up whatever lies in the paths of the trawls. Any turtles, fish, and other marine species swept up in the nets are considered unprofitable "by-catch" and are generally deposited — dead — back into the ocean.'

The typical ratio for by-catch is about 10 to 1 in tropical areas; the shrimp industry is responsible for about a third of the world total. The impact of the industry is only getting worse as the amount of fishing increases. China, for example, which takes the most shrimp of any country in the world, doubled its take between 1990 and 2000, to 1.089 million tonnes.

Unfortunately, farmed shrimp and prawns are not good for the environment, either. The waste the farms produce, from fertilisers and chemicals used to kill bugs in the water, usually ends up in waterways and estuaries and is often dumped straight into the ocean. Prawn farming has also caused tremendous habitat destruction, usually in Third World countries and particularly in Thailand and Vietnam. Nearly one quarter of the world's remaining tropical mangrove forests were destroyed during the past two decades — largely to make way for shrimp farms. Traditional, often sustainable, ways of life are destroyed. The Indian physicist and environmental advocate Vandana Shiva has estimated that while the average shrimp farm provides about 15 jobs on the farm and a further 50 security jobs, it takes away the land and traditional lifestyle of 50,000 people.

Not all of the news is gloomy. There are some species, like Chinese carp, oysters and green-lipped mussels, that are well suited to aquaculture and are being farmed highly successfully. Why are these fish different from salmon or prawns and shrimp? They are filter feeders, passing thousands of litres of seawater over efficient nutrient extractors. They will concentrate every nasty bug in the water in which they are raised and render themselves a health hazard if they are grown in anything but the purest water. They do not need antibiotics because they have always lived in enormous colonies, and the farmers of these delicacies have merely replicated nature's conditions.

Led by New Zealand, many countries are beginning to establish extensive marine reserves where no fishing is permitted. These areas effectively become breeding grounds for many types of fish, seeding sustainable fisheries in surrounding areas. New Zealand has 31 reserves, and is aiming to have 10 to 20 per cent of its coastal waters protected in the near future.

Finally, much is being made of a new style of fish and prawn farming referred to as 'organic', which uses much lower population densities and conforms to higher environmental standards. While there are still quite a few problems to iron out, we watch the evolution of this industry with hope.

It is not unreasonable to demand that future generations have the right to catch and eat fish in moderation, and that our decision-makers must take all the necessary steps to ensure this — with a decent margin for error. It is sobering to read that in the latter stages of the exploitation of the great auk, the penalty in England for possessing any part of the bird was a public whipping, but the law was enacted too late to save it. When we start the public whippings of the new era, perhaps the functionaries who use public relations-speak to say that 'Everything's all right' will be top of the list.

STRATEGY 21 BUY ONLY 'GREEN' FISH'

Download a fisheries guide from one of the websites we have listed, and buy only the less threatened species. Look for organic-farmed options and support the formation of marine reserves.

This is the last strategy that we have written as such. Most of the actions in Chapter 7 require individualised, professional advice. The strategies we recommend in Part Three of this book are summarised in Chapter 13.

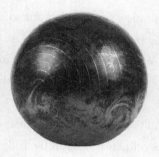

7 | eat your medicine

An introduction to nutritional medicine

jackie   A wonderful colleague from my obstetric days, Carolyn Young, would often comment on how my energy and zest through late-night deliveries must have come from way too much health food as a child. She was right! My childhood was full of simple food: lots of unadulterated vegetables, sandwiches packed with greens that we fondly named 'hedge sandwiches', fruit, nuts, and never a dressing or sauce in sight. This came from my parents: my father's insatiable pursuit of health and energy for his sport, and my mother's desire to maintain her youthful figure. These early lessons have stuck with me throughout my life.

Once I had trained as a doctor and finished my years in the hospital system, I completed advanced studies in nutritional medicine and obstetrics. For the next 13 years I practiced obstetrics, in awe of the powerful process of pregnancy, childbirth and parenting. Political change eventually forced me, and the majority of New Zealand GPs, out of obstetric practice. This meant the loss of a wonderful service for women in New Zealand, but for me it resulted in a shift of focus back to nutritional medicine.

I have always seen medicine as a forum to promote health rather than medication, and believe that with knowledge and motivation people can change their habits to live more fulfilled lives through exercise and good nutrition. In 2003, I was fortunate enough to find a group of like-minded professionals and joined the Holistic Medical Centre (HMC) in Auckland as a general practitioner.

Our philosophy is simple: vital health for our patients. The current healthcare model defines health as the lack of symptoms. Our definition reaches far beyond this. We believe that a deeper understanding is required of the factors that promote dynamic, robust health or, conversely, foster ill health.

By taking a close look at the complex biochemistry of an individual and the workings of the body at a cellular level, and by finding what is needed for full function and what disease or pathology occurs when nutrients are missing, we can begin to understand how nutrients, hormones, neurotransmitters and lifestyle factors can support vitality. A balanced, enriched biochemical environment is fertile ground for the creation of healthy cells.

In our practice at HMC we combine this nutritional medicine with orthodox medical training and appropriate prescribing of 21st century medicines in an approach known as integrated medicine. Integrated medicine views health not merely as the absence of symptoms, but as a realm that incorporates well-being, good sleep, a clear and calm mind, wonderful energy and a happy life force. We believe that, in the words of Louis Pasteur: 'The internal milieu of the body needs to be in homeostasis [balance] and this in itself creates a form of disease prevention.'

In our view, clinicians should be committed to achieving real improvements in pain management, treatment of illness and quality of life for their patients. Exhausting the known treatment approaches or suppressing symptoms is simply not enough. It is essential as a practitioner to always look for the cause of illness and to be committed to getting results. We would be happy to see the same principle applied to healthcare that exists for many other service industries — that is, being paid for results.

At HMC we see nutritional deficiency every day. We don't often see scurvy, rickets or beriberi, which are the severe forms of nutrient deficiency, but many common disorders and diseases can be cured by adding simple nutrients into our diet. We must therefore acknowledge that diet has a direct effect on health. We also know that people have very different nutritional needs. We don't advocate general supplementation for everyone. We believe that with appropriate testing it is possible to identify vitamin deficiency in individuals and combat this with targeted nutrition and supplementation.

The food we eat is often grown under conditions designed to enhance yield and shelf life, rather than to improve our health and well-being. It is grown in nutrient-poor soil, then overly processed and preserved. If we look at the actual nutrient content of our food, it is often lacking in the essential vitamins, minerals, oils and proteins that maintain and repair our bodies.

The knowledge and case studies on the following pages come from the work we do at HMC. Some may seem unbelievable to you. We've been surprised ourselves at times by the immediate impact nutritional medicine can have. It's important to keep in mind that everything we discuss is considered in the context of years of study and training as orthodox medical professionals.

It is impossible to do justice to such an important and vast subject as nutritional medicine in one chapter of a book, but we would like to pass on some of our experiences. We've selected just a few of the areas in which we have found nutritional medicine to be particularly effective. Our examples are not designed to be prescriptive because treatment is individualised and associated with appropriate blood, saliva, urine and hair testing. As with all things medical, we issue the caution that a little bit of knowledge can be dangerous. I encourage you to read more and find someone in your town or city who can help you with any specific issues you are facing. We hope that you will be inspired to venture further into this amazing world!

(Please note that because biochemistry is such a complex subject, some of the scientific processes described below have been simplified for the purposes of this book.)

Depression (and other mood disorders)

In many cases, if the body has the right raw materials it will get along just fine. Our diagnosis often involves understanding what materials are missing.

We treat a large number of people with 'depression'. We usually begin by improving their energy levels, promoting sufficient uninterrupted sleep, correcting low vitamin D and ensuring that their diet contains adequate protein. In the great majority of cases, this is all that's required.

It's extremely common to find that there is a history of stress and fatigue or exhaustion before the mood-related problems arise. When someone is exhausted, it's very difficult for them to feel happy and positive, and conversely it's difficult for a person who has plenty of energy to feel down. If sufficient vitamin D and amino acids (from protein) are available, then the raw materials are present for the synthesis of melatonin for sleep, and of mood-stabilising neurotransmitters such as serotonin, dopamine, noradrenalin and vasopressin.

This is vastly different from the traditional medical model that does not have a treatment for exhaustion. Many people are given anti-depressant medication following periods of stress and subsequent exhaustion.

CASE STUDY 1

A 50-year-old woman came to us with low mood and ideas of suicide. When we tested her vitamin D it was very low. Within a week of prescription vitamin D her mood was lifted and all suicidal thoughts had gone.

Anti-depressant medication

Anti-depressant medication is now widely used in orthodox medicine. The most common form is selective serotonin reuptake inhibitors (SSRIs), which increase levels of the mood-elevating hormone serotonin. What patients are rarely told, however, is how hard it is to withdraw from these drugs, and the serious side effects they may cause. When side effects do occur, often the dose is increased or another medication is added.

This does not happen to everyone, but on a daily basis at HMC we are helping someone cope with the side effects or withdrawal effects of anti-depressants. We actually feel so strongly about the negative effects of anti-depressants that we have a policy not to prescribe this class of drugs.

Despite current medical dogma on the subject, we see it like this: we have clearly observed side effects like insomnia with SSRI anti-depressant medication. We have scoured medical literature for information about why this is so and can find little by way of satisfactory explanation. If, however, we observe that an overwhelming number of patients on anti-depressants complain of insomnia after starting their medication, then we have empirical *evidence* — not anecdote. If medical literature does not appear to provide evidence to support a regular clinical observation such as ours, this does not mean that it cannot be observed as a truth.

CASE STUDY 2

A boy of 15 years came to us with his parents. He barely spoke and his parents described him as having absolutely no energy; he was unable to attend school or leave the house. Making even the smallest decision was completely overwhelming for him. The boy seemed unable to smile and interaction with his very concerned family was minimal. Interestingly, he also had terribly disturbed sleep.

He had had surgery following a car accident two years earlier. Morphine and Tramadol, which were used for pain relief after the surgery, can have some side effects such as depression and hallucinations, which are normally temporary. However, this boy had been put on anti-depressant and anti-psychotic medication and had steadily become more withdrawn.

Initially, we gave him some magnesium to assist sleep and B vitamins to aid his energy. When we reviewed his blood tests we found he had the lowest vitamin D levels we had ever seen!

His vitamin D was 19 µg/l (micrograms per litre); it should have been in the range of 100–150. This deficiency causes very low mood and sleep problems. We gave him high-quality prescription vitamin D to correct this.

His blood tests also revealed some auto-antibody activity,

which we know creates fatigue. To counter that, we gave him coenzyme Q10 (CoQ10), zinc and selenium.

The following week his psychiatrist halved his anti-psychotic medication. Two weeks later the boy was much brighter. He was talking, smiling and even making jokes. We asked him to tell us what his energy levels were like and he said 6/10, an improvement from 3/10 before coming to see us. After further consultation with the psychiatrist, we stopped the anti-psychotic medication altogether.

We slowly decreased his anti-depressant medication (as there are frequently side effects when people stop taking anti-depressants) and a few months later he was medication-free, totally well, full of energy and back at school!

Correcting low vitamin D levels, and prescribing appropriate doses of magnesium and sometimes melatonin, can provide a dramatic improvement in the quality of sleep for those taking SSRI medication or wanting to withdraw from it. The doses of melatonin and magnesium we use often have to be increased to aid in the sometimes severe insomnia encountered when withdrawing from the medication. However, if vitamin D levels are kept between 100 and 150 µg/l, and high doses of magnesium and B vitamins are given with appropriate doses of melatonin, the withdrawal effects should be minimal.

Common minor side effects when withdrawing from these medications are sensations of electric shock and anxiety. These should disappear with high doses of magnesium.

Mood maintenance through healthy nutrition

There are a number of dietary elements that can help protect us against the factors that commonly lead to depression. At the top of this list is an adequate intake of of high-quality protein.

As mentioned above, our bodies make mood-affecting neurotransmitters or hormones from amino acids that come from protein. It is startling to us how many people's blood tests show them to be protein-deficient, especially women! A diet of toast and cereal for breakfast, sandwiches for lunch and a muffin in the afternoon will be familiar to many of you. This diet means there is minimal protein until dinnertime. Eating enough protein helps stabilise blood sugars, provides consistent energy levels and assists in weight stabilisation. Also, the individual amino acids that make up protein are crucial to the way the body functions.

The following is a description of some of the key neurotransmitters/ hormones required for the maintenance of mood and the food sources that provide us with amino acids and other building blocks. Put simply, eat enough of the right protein sources throughout the day and you'll have the best chance of staying happy and healthy.

It would be really helpful if Hollywood could push home this message. Next time the heroine in a romantic comedy has an emotional meltdown and goes for the chocolate cookies, she should stop and say: 'No, it's walnuts I need right now!'

Serotonin

Serotonin is the main neurotransmitter associated with mood. Low serotonin is associated with depression, anxiety, aggressiveness and attention deficit hyperactivity disorder (ADHD). The most common anti-depressant prescribed by doctors blocks the breakdown of this substance in an effort to alleviate depression.

For our bodies to manufacture serotonin we require adequate levels of tryptophan, vitamin B6 and folate.

- *Tryptophan* is an amino acid that is present in high levels in meat, pumpkin, spirulina and soy. (Stick to traditionally prepared soy products such as miso, tempeh, tofu and soy milk to avoid health risks posed by overconsumption of modern industrial soy products.) Tryptophan is also important in the production of melatonin (see below), and in immune system and antioxidant functions.

- *Vitamin B6* (pyridoxine) is found in beef, walnuts, bananas, spinach, sunflower seeds, eggs, fish, chicken, brewer's yeast and salmon. (Try to source wild or organic salmon to avoid some of the health risks of farmed salmon and the environmental damage caused by salmon farming — see previous chapter.) B6 is involved in more body functions than almost any other nutrient, affecting both mental and physical health.

- *Folate* is considered a brain food. It's found in brewer's yeast, most types of beans and peas, beef and lamb (especially grass-fed organic meat), liver, eggs, brown rice and other whole grains, sunflower seeds and particularly in green leafy vegetables such as kale and spinach. It is needed for energy production, healthy cell replication, protein metabolism and the formation of red and white blood cells. Folate is vital in pregnancy as it ensures the correct development of nerve cells, preventing spina bifida and anencephaly.

Our bodies cannot make serotonin without the presence of these three basic materials.

Melatonin

Melatonin is made from serotonin and is the hormone responsible for setting our body's night and day rhythm. It is needed for deep, restful sleep. Waking during the night or restless, light sleeping patterns often indicate low levels of melatonin. It is made in the brain and stored during the day by the action of sunlight on the skin and eyes. Sunlight is also known to increase serotonin and vitamin D levels.

We know you look great in your sunglasses, but if you have sleep problems we suggest you use them only when you really need them. Melatonin *release* is stimulated by twilight on your naked eyes so again, how about stopping to watch some beautiful sunsets without those groovy glasses.

We often prescribe supplemental melatonin to help people experiencing exhaustion and disrupted sleep to regain a normal cycle and a better mood.

CASE STUDY 3

We recently saw a 57-year-old man who had been under stress, sleeping poorly for two years, and had developed progressively lower energy levels. Three mg of melatonin at night for a month helped get him back into a regular sleeping

pattern and feeling good. (In this rejuvenated state he was able to deal with the root cause of the problem by making some life decisions that reduced his stress levels.)

This is a great example of how different facets of a person's life can contribute to their feeling poorly. Until he had the energy to face his issues, this man was in a vicious cycle of not sleeping properly because he was stressed, which gave him less energy, which meant he wasn't dealing with life matters that led to more stress!

Vasopressin

Vasopressin is another hormone that is important for deep sleep, as well as memory, learning, concentration, blood pressure regulation and preventing dehydration. This interesting hormone is made up of nine amino acids, which are available from a wide range of protein-rich foods. Alcohol and caffeine reduce our secretion of vasopressin.

It's not news that caffeine keeps us awake and most of us know about alcohol impairing our memory. Less is best.

Dopamine

Dopamine is a neurotransmitter that is vital for mood and libido. It is also associated with Parkinson's, Alzheimer's, ADHD and menstrual problems in women.

Dopamine is used in the synthesis of adrenaline, so it is not surprising that those who experience long-term stress show symptoms of dopamine deficiency. This usually creates a diminished ability to experience pleasure. To make dopamine we need vitamin B6 and tyrosine.

- The amino acid *tyrosine* is found in high levels in soy, meat, spirulina, yoghurt, peanut butter and tuna. (Don't eat *blue fin* tuna; it's an endangered species that often contains high levels of mercury and other toxins.) Tyrosine is also synthesised from phenylalanine. The best food sources of phenylalanine are fermented soy products, meat, fish and spirulina.

Noradrenalin

Noradrenalin is made in the adrenal glands, which sit on top of the kidneys. It is a hormone in the blood and a neurotransmitter in the nervous system, and is made from dopamine. Noradrenalin is essential for mood, energy, alertness, memory and the production of melatonin. To make noradrenalin we need tyrosine, phenylalanine, vitamin B6 and vitamin C.

So how can you eat the right amount of protein? Here are a few practical suggestions for building into your diet the proteins and vitamins required for mood maintenance:

- Eat protein with every meal — and trust me, a cheese sandwich won't cut it! Ideal sources are eggs, fish, meat, chicken, tofu and tempeh (fermented soy products) and nuts.

- Try using ground almonds instead of flour in your baking. Our daughter adds rice protein powder into her baking as a way to help her partner get sufficient protein for his active lifestyle.

- Legumes such as lentils and chickpeas need to be combined with nuts and seeds to boost protein levels.

- For breakfast, try sardines on toast (and get the added energy benefits of CoQ10), tuna or an egg — or a tablespoon of nuts or almond butter in your smoothie.

- Lunch could be a lamb/tuna/tofu/egg salad with one of the many nut-based sauces available, such as cashew and coriander pesto.

- Rice-based protein powders are great for people sensitive to dairy and soy.

- It's good to include raw nuts in your snacks.

Here's a superb smoothie recipe from Bill Robertson (Les Mills International's Australian agent):

250 ml water

250 ml milk (cow's, goat's, rice, almond) or more water

2 tsp lecithin granules

2 tbsp LSA (linseed, sunflower, almonds), available at health food stores

3 tbsp unsweetened yoghurt

1 tbsp flaxseed oil

1 or 2 eggs

1 banana

½–1 cup berries (blueberries, raspberries, blackberries)

Mix for one minute or so, and enjoy as your breakfast or lunch..

Exhaustion or adrenal fatigue

Profound exhaustion or burnout can be indistinguishable from the symptoms of clinical depression. These symptoms include fatigue, disturbed sleep, lack of enjoyment, lethargy and anxiety. Nutritionally speaking, burnout and exhaustion are very simple to treat, and dealing with them appropriately will provide the desired outcome without putting the 'depression' label on the medical records.

Adrenal fatigue is another term to describe exhaustion, more commonly used by naturopaths than doctors. The use of this term stems from the naturopathic belief that exhaustion occurs when the adrenal glands produce too much of the so-called stress hormones over too long a period of time.

The adrenal gland hormones, which include adrenaline, noradrenalin, cortisol, pregnenolone and DHEA, are very important for energy, mood, mental alertness, restful sleep, immunity and the production of male and female hormones. Problems with this gland can therefore create various and seemingly unrelated problems.

Under stress, the adrenal glands produce a large amount of adrenaline and cortisol. Many people are familiar with the feeling of running on nervous energy that is often associated with this. The theory is that problems begin to occur when this continues over a sustained period of time and the adrenal glands begin to become fatigued. A reliance on coffee and other stimulants can develop, and these begin to have a lessened effect.

A person with adrenal fatigue typically experiences symptoms like tiredness not relieved by sleeping, waking between 1 and 4 am, heart palpitations from adrenaline surges (especially when resting) and anxiety. Falling asleep is not usually a problem due to extreme tiredness. Some people experience more frequent infections and if the exhaustion has been sustained, there can be problems with the male and female hormones.

In the absence of other diagnoses such as anaemia or cardiovascular disease these people are often prescribed anti-depressants, as doctors sometimes do not seem to know how to treat simple exhaustion!

Blood tests are important in diagnosing the condition. It's necessary to check levels of cortisol, DHEA, Vitamin D, thyroid hormones, vitamin B12 and folate, and do full blood count, liver function, full iron and auto-antibody studies. (Auto-antibodies can be treated and have a significant effect on energy levels. Simply explained, auto-antibodies occur when the body mistakenly starts to attack itself.)

In order to fully treat exhaustion, vitamin, mineral and sometimes herbal supplements are required for two to three months. However energy levels can be increased substantially within several days. If you liken your body to a car, as soon as you refill the tank it goes again. It won't run perfectly until it has a good tune-up, but it will run much better than when there's no gas at all.

CASE STUDY 4

We recently had a 24-year-old woman visit our clinic who had taken a month off work due to grief, anxiety, depression and fatigue. She was sleeping 12 hours a day. Her GP had proposed anti-depressants, but a counsellor suggested a natural approach. After two weeks of nutritional help, her fatigue, depression and grief had lifted and she was back at work. We're not suggesting that grief can be 'cured', but there are ways of maintaining the

balance within your body during times of intense grief to help you cope.

CASE STUDY 5

A 51-year-old woman came to us in November 2006 suffering fatigue, depression and recurring illness. In the early 1990s she had experienced burnout from her job and other stresses, and every month since had suffered from what she described as colds and flu. In her words: 'My first appointment here at the Holistic Centre was marvellous because my experience was clearly familiar to them . . . After tests and full interviews with a naturopath and doctor, by January I felt 7/10 instead of 3/10, had lost five kilos and was looking for full-time work.'

In addition to the vitamins, minerals and herbal supplements we've listed above, two supplements we sometimes use in treating exhaustion are DHEA and pregnenolone. We use them in other clinical settings, too.

DHEA

DHEA, as noted above, is one of the hormones produced by the adrenal glands. It is extremely important to our health and when we have been under stress for long periods of time, its production can decrease. It is a strong antioxidant (so is favoured by anti-ageing practitioners) and is very beneficial to the immune system. It has been shown to be protective against many forms of cancer. DHEA also improves energy and is very useful in the treatment of depression and anxiety. Blood tests are needed to determine levels in the body and it can be prescribed as a supplement. We believe that levels over four µmol/l are optimal.

We always start prescribing small doses of hormones. We only use those that are bio-identical i.e. absolutely the same as those made in our bodies. We very finely adjust the dose, as dictated by each individual's health and ongoing blood test results.

CASE STUDY 6

A very healthy 75-year-old man came to us complaining of low energy levels. He had exercised regularly and been a committed vegetarian almost all his life. But despite being in outwardly excellent shape, he had recently started to feel very low. His blood tests revealed DHEA levels of almost zero! A very small supplement made a huge difference, restoring his energy levels and making a big improvement to his life.

Here was a man who would most probably have been given anti-depressants under conventional medicine, with all the troubling side effects.

Pregnenolone

Pregnenolone is often called the grandmother hormone, as it is necessary for the production of many other hormones, such as estrogens, testosterone, DHEA, cortisol and progesterone. It is made predominantly in the adrenal glands, so keeping these glands working well is important. Pregnenolone is critical for memory, and low levels are associated with anxiety, depression and Alzheimer's. We find it useful for menopausal woman who are under a lot of stress and are experiencing anxiety and 'fuzzy-headedness'. A small supplement helps these women to produce the appropriate hormones they need.

Interestingly, pregnenolone is made from cholesterol. In individuals with low cholesterol levels there can be a corresponding deficiency in other hormones, such as testosterone. We often see this see in people on cholesterol-lowering drugs, another class of medication we believe is over-prescribed, and so we avoid these drugs in favour of natural treatments.

The chart below shows the pathways in the production of these hormones. Note the importance of cholesterol, pregnenolone and DHEA in the formation of so many other hormones. E1, E2 and E3 are the three types of estrogen in our bodies.

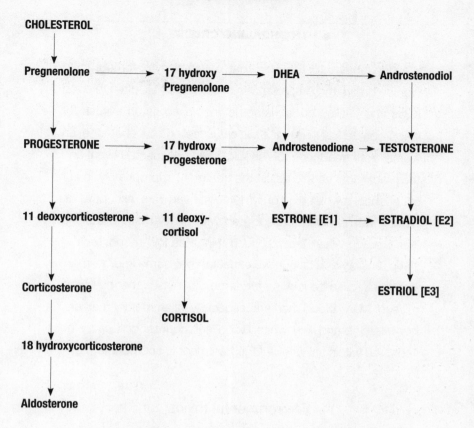

Depression — summary

The number of people currently experiencing depression tells us there are underlying problems that need to be addressed in our society. However, it is impossible to underestimate the importance of good food and sound sleep. Just ensuring these two things are okay will provide wonderful results for most patients.

It is important to note that plenty of convalescence after illness or significant stressful events is extremely important, as is expert psychological counselling when required. Too often, people push themselves too hard after a stressful event and subsequently suffer. We also frequently prescribe exercise, which, as we discussed in Chapter 4, can play a very effective part in treating depression.

If you're on anti-depressants it's not a great idea to flush them away, but it's well worth finding an expert who can help you withdraw from them safely and ensure that your body's nutritional and biochemical needs are being met.

● 'THE HEALING CRISIS'

We don't buy into the idea that patients' symptoms should worsen before they improve. We believe that this, often referred to as 'the healing crisis', is sometimes used as an excuse for inappropriate treatment. If a patient is feeling no better, or even worse, from treatment, this should be an unexpected event and the practitioner should adjust the treatment appropriately. In our experience, a worsening of symptoms is very rare, except when dealing with problems associated with heavy metal poisoning (see below). When treating such things as low mood, lack of sleep, anxiety and fatigue we expect to see some improvement in a week, or to be looking for some other issue that has been missed. Many blood markers, especially inflammatory markers, low vitamins and low white blood cell counts, can easily be improved within six weeks if the treatment is appropriate.

Environmental toxins

Another problem of modern society is environmental toxins. Millions of people a year die from the effects of air, water, food and soil pollution. Because of their size, physiology and behaviour, children are most at risk. The World Health Organization states that *three million* children die every year as a result of pollution. Cleaning up the environment is one of the many issues we need to address in order to create a better world for them.

Heavy metal poisoning is caused by environmental factors. Here are some examples of how integrated medicine can help to undo some of the damage.

Heavy metal poisoning

Heavy metals are a major category of toxins that pose a significant threat to health through occupational and environmental exposure. Lead and mercury are the most toxic, closely followed by arsenic and cadmium. Both lead and mercury are capable of exerting toxic effects at very low levels of exposure. They can be inhaled, ingested or absorbed through the skin, as is the case with lead. If they are not excreted, they can be sequestered in relatively high concentrations by some organs, for many years — silent and potentially dangerous.

Doctors who study environmental medicine are well aware of the impact that heavy metals can have on health. The types of symptoms that lead us to suspect problems with heavy metals are: a chronically low white blood cell count, auto-antibodies, significantly decreased mental clarity, memory problems, fatigue, depression, an under-active thyroid gland and unexplained neurological symptoms such as numbness, pain, tingling and tremor. All of these symptoms should be thoroughly investigated from a medical point of view initially, to eliminate other possible causes.

Miners, metal workers, ceramic workers, dentists and dental technicians are regularly exposed to heavy metals. The use of lead-based paints (especially marine paints) and renovating old houses containing those paints is also dangerous. Cigarette smoking exposes people to cadmium, arsenic, mercury and lead, as well as other toxic substances.

Lead

During the 20th century more people were exposed to lead than ever before. Lead poisoning gained widespread public attention when children were found to have been poisoned by chips of lead-based paint peeling off walls, or by playing in lead-contaminated dirt. Many of these sources are still common in our environment today. Even low-level exposure was found to be associated with impaired intellectual development and behavioural problems. Studies have shown that a person's IQ falls by up to six points for every ten micrograms of lead per decilitre of blood (μg/dl). The majority of children living in cities where leaded gasoline is still permitted have been shown to have blood lead levels above this (WHO statistics).

Lead exposure can also cause anaemia, kidney disease, hearing damage and impaired fertility; at high levels, it can result in coma or death.

Mercury

Mercury is even more toxic than lead. Environmental exposure to mercury takes place most commonly through eating contaminated fish or breathing in vapour generated by ordinary dental amalgam fillings. The mercury preservative thiomersal is still used in a number of vaccines. Mercury is also in a wide variety of everyday products: cosmetics, fabric softeners, latex, plastics, polishes, solvents, ink used by printers and tattooists, and wood preservatives. If you were a baby in the 1940s or earlier you may have had a teething powder containing mercury that could cause Pink Disease (acrodynia).

Our body's natural mechanism for removing heavy metals is a group of proteins called metallothioneins (MTs), which are also involved in the development of brain cells and synaptic connections. Once bound within MTs, toxic metals become relatively harmless. The affinity of MTs (which means their ability to bind to the metals) for mercury is especially powerful, so mercury can be removed from the body.

The highest levels of MTs are found in the intestinal mucosa in the gut, forming a barrier to mercury, lead, cadmium and other heavy metals. In healthy people, ingested metal toxins are bound in mucosal MT, which is excreted by the body harmlessly every 5–10 days in the stool.

These vitally important proteins are made from other nutrients. The nutrients required for the manufacture of MT proteins are zinc, two forms of vitamin B6 (pyridoxal-5-phosphate and pyridoxine hydrochloride), selenium, manganese, vitamins C and E, and 14 different amino acids. As long as these nutrients are present there is a certain amount of protection against metals that are ingested orally, such as those found in fish.

Sulphur has a strong affinity for heavy metals (especially for mercury) so it is another important nutrient to protect us from heavy metals. Sulphur is found in Brussels sprouts, cabbage, kale, garlic, onions, fish, turnips and wheat germ.

Chlorella is another useful nutrient to assist in the removal of heavy metals. We use it with DMSA (dimercaptosuccinic acid, a common sulphur-based chelating agent) because it contains many amino acids and helps form the MTs.

Some people have a genetic weakness in their ability to handle heavy metals in comparison to other people. This can be measured in a blood test that shows genetic tissue typing called Apolipoprotein E (Apo E) genotyping. This protein is made up of 29 amino acids and its structure is an indicator of the risk of developing Alzheimer's. We can't change this genotype but it helps us in assessing the whole picture of a person's symptoms and blood test results. Then, if necessary, we can recommend a urinary metal test. If toxic metals show in this test we plan an appropriate detoxification.

To test for metals we use DMSA. This chelating agent is in capsule form and assists in drawing heavy metals out of the tissue and into the blood. Chelating agents bind metals into stable compounds with low toxicity and enhance their excretion from the body.

In the provocation test, DMSA is taken orally. Urine is then collected over a six-hour period and sent away to be measured for 15 different heavy metals. Mercury and lead are by far the most commonly elevated. Sometimes we also use DMSA as part of the detoxification protocol.

This test is required if heavy metal exposure is to be confirmed. Blood tests only show recent exposure.

CASE STUDY

In 2006 we had a 44-year-old man come to visit us with joint pains in his wrists, knees, ankles and fingers; depression and anxiety; problems with mental fog; and odd, unexplained pains in differing parts of the body, sometimes sharp, sometimes dull. He also had a metallic taste in his mouth. At night he would get numbness and tingling in his arms and legs (whole limb) and his fine-motor skills were decreasing. He had been on Prozac in the past and as a result of the new symptoms. He had been to many doctors but still felt that he was getting worse.

His blood tests revealed auto-antibodies and a low white blood cell count (specifically neutrophils). He commented that his doctors had noted this in his blood tests on many occasions but were only monitoring it.

A couple of interesting things stood out from our initial discussions about his history. This man had a mouth full of very large, old amalgam fillings and he had worked on houses

years ago which had exposed him to lead-based paints. He had also worked with ceramics that had exposed him to thallium.

We recommended he see a dentist who specialised in the safe removal of amalgam fillings and had these replaced with composite (white) fillings. He decided he wanted to do the provocation urine test with DMSA to see for himself if metals were truly the problem.

Tellingly, when he took the DMSA (which is only two capsules), the neurological symptoms and the metal taste in his mouth completely disappeared for a time and he felt temporarily very well. As suspected, the urine test showed high levels of lead, mercury and thallium.

He is currently following a heavy metal detoxification programme. He was amazed on three counts: firstly, that the blood tests confirmed our suspicions; secondly, how well he felt while the DMSA had drawn the metals into his bloodstream; and thirdly, that it had taken so long for him to find relief. And his relief was two-fold: he finally knew what was causing his pain and unusual symptoms, and he was experiencing ever-improving health.

CASE STUDY 8

We treated a woman who had suffered from severe Ménière's disease (an inner ear disorder that can affect hearing and balance) for years, needing large amounts of medication. Symptoms of the disease include vertigo, spinning sensations, severe vomiting and hearing loss as well as sometimes only being able to hear a sound similar to a fire alarm in one's head. It can be a very debilitating condition.

We tested for heavy metals and it turned out that our patient had high levels of mercury in her urine. We recommended that she have her old amalgam fillings removed and replaced with composite fillings. She was gradually improving, but while one quadrant of her mouth was being treated she had the worst Ménière's attack that she had experienced for a long time. She recovered, completed the fillings removal and is now completely well. No more Ménière's.

CASE STUDY 9

A woman we saw recently suffered from the skin disease lichen planus. The condition had been getting worse and she was now experiencing aches throughout her body. She had found no medical specialists who were able to help her.

When we applied the provocation test with DMSA, the aches disappeared temporarily and she felt good. The blood test for Apo E genotype showed she only had 50 per cent genetic protection against heavy metals. Based on these findings we advised her to see a dentist specialising in the removal of amalgams. When he tested the fillings they showed a very high reading, which indicated that the mercury was unstable. She also took a urine test, which showed levels of heavy metals in her body. The test results found elevated levels of tungsten, mercury and lead. After complete replacement of the mercury fillings with composite fillings and a detoxification with DMSA, the lichen planus disappeared.

CASE STUDY 10

A woman in her 60s had problems with an under-active thyroid gland for many years. She also had thyroid antibodies, which meant her immune system was attacking her thyroid and gradually decreasing its ability to function. We put her on an iodine supplement (which helps with the production of the thyroid hormone thyroxine) as well as zinc and selenium (they assist in the production of thyroxine but coincidentally help with the removal of heavy metals). These nutrients did improve

the production of thyroid hormone but did little to stem the problem with the auto-antibodies. We suggested that the best thing she could do for her thyroid health was to have her amalgam fillings replaced with white ones, but did not expect her to follow through on our recommendation. To our delight (and hers) she did have this done and her thyroid blood results normalised for the first time in years. She continued with supplements and the thyroid results began to take on an overactive picture! She removed the supplements for her thyroid, and her thyroid function tests corrected fully. We have a very medical term for this kind of result: wow.

If you would like more information on heavy metals, a great deal of research (especially with regard to mental health) has been conducted by a committed group of doctors at the Pfeiffer Institute: *www.hriptc.org*.

Asthma

Asthma is a common condition of the lungs that is characterised by increased responsiveness of the airways to many stimuli e.g. dust mites, cold air, exercise, viral infections, irritants such as pollens, animal hair, certain foods and drugs and, again, environmental pollution. It involves an inflammatory response, which causes a thickening in the airways due to an excess production of mucous, and contraction of the muscles in the airways of the lungs (bronchospasm).

The following are two nutritional approaches we have used successfully in treating asthma. We also address any food sensitivities.

Magnesium

The practical application of knowledge in biochemistry and nutritional biochemistry can provide startling results for patients. Magnesium, a mineral, is used in building bones, manufacturing proteins, releasing energy from muscle storage and regulating body temperature. It is well known for alleviating muscle cramps in skeletal muscle, but it also appears to do this in smooth muscle e.g. the airways in the lungs and blood vessel walls.

When there is a magnesium deficiency, more calcium is contained within the muscle cells, which increases their ability to contract. Magnesium displaces calcium from muscle cell surfaces, therefore effectively relaxing the muscles in the blood vessel walls, and causes a widening of the blood vessels (vasodilation), which drops blood pressure and relieves spasm in the airways of the lungs. This is really important in conditions like hypertension (high blood pressure) and asthma — the broncho-constrictive aspect of this condition.

We tried potent practitioner-only magnesium on our asthmatic patients to see if it lessened their need for Ventolin (salbutamol), the drug that reduces muscle spasm in the lungs. This has repeatedly worked very well.

It is very difficult to eat enough magnesium in the average modern diet. The richest food sources are pumpkin seeds, Brazil nuts, halibut, almonds, cashews, parsnips, brewer's yeast, spinach, various beans and peas, various whole grains and molasses. Much magnesium is also lost in cooking. It's no wonder that many of our children experience asthma when it's raw spinach, beans, whole grains and molasses that help keep it at bay.

Omega-3

It is well known that omega-3 oils produce anti-inflammatory prostaglandins in the body, so we suspected they would be of benefit in reducing the inflammatory aspect of asthma. This also worked very well, with the correct doses. An initial dose of 6000 mg daily for adults is ideal.

Fish oil is far superior to other oils when reducing inflammation and pain because it is rapidly incorporated into the body's tissues. Plant-based sources can be used, but the process is much slower and less efficient. Small-fish sources such as sardines and anchovies are healthier and more ecologically sound. Farmed salmon in the southern hemisphere has lower risks than in the northern hemisphere, owing to our lower levels of pollution, but as explained in Chapter 6, all farmed salmon has health risks and wild salmon is not currently a sustainable food source for mass consumption.

CASE STUDY 11

We have been treating asthmatics in this way with great success. One notable case is a 40-year-old woman who had

asthma since childhood. Twice a day she would take inhaled steroids and Ventolin, and every year would need several courses of prednisone (oral steroids) to get her though the winter. It was common for her to be so sick that she would spend a week in hospital every year.

We started her on practitioner-only magnesium and omega-3. After two months she slowly started to reduce her medications. (We always advocate staying on regular medications until a patient is symptom-free. Even then, a reduction should be slow and guided.) Two years later this lively woman takes no medication other than her nutritional supplements, and we only see her when she comes to collect them! She has had no prednisone and no hospital admissions since she started with us. This has made a huge positive change to her life.

CASE STUDY 12

An asthmatic pre-school brother and sister we saw last year are now medication-free following the introduction of magnesium and omega-3 to their diets. They were both allergic to dairy foods and monosodium glutamate (MSG). Taking these out of their diets has transformed their health and growth. (Various foods seem to set off an asthmatic reaction in certain individuals. Dairy foods appear to be the most common culprit. If dairy is not the problem, it can often be wheat and potatoes.)

These are just two of *numerous* examples of our patients who now live with much better lung function and reduced or no asthma medication as a result of supplementation with magnesium and omega-3 fish oils.

These two powerful nutrients are also useful in the treatment of many other conditions.

● THE MAGIC OF MAGNESIUM

Magnesium and hypertension

There are many studies that link low magnesium levels and high blood pressure. People can even have normal levels of magnesium on blood tests, but have low levels in their tissues. It is reported that 50 per cent of magnesium-depleted people have hypertension, and that their blood pressure returns to normal with supplementation. This effect may take three to six months, but patients are often relieved to use this simple approach in preference to experiencing the side effects of medication.

CASE STUDY 13

I recently treated a delightful young man who was determined not to take medication for his raised blood pressure. After three months of magnesium supplementation and, of course, some good old exercise, his blood pressure was a little on the low side of normal!

CASE STUDY 14

One of my most inspiring patients is 82 and has energy I hope to have at her age. She has been able to significantly reduce her medications by using magnesium. After suffering from hypertension for 50 years despite medication, she always has a good laugh at how normal her blood pressure is now because of magnesium supplementation.

Magnesium and headaches

Based on the idea that headaches and migraines (those that lack a serious organic cause) are related to vasoconstriction or the contraction of muscles in the blood vessel walls, we wondered if magnesium, again, would be clinically useful. We have had wonderful results. We have found that appropriate magnesium supplementation results in improvements for almost all patients suffering from chronic headaches. Many people report 100 per cent improvement. Imagine moving from years of debilitating headaches, to within weeks having none at all! Magnesium

> The fourth highest cause of death in the US is from iatrogenic causes, i.e. the side effects of medicine!

is very important for tension headaches, vascular headaches and stress headaches, and is also useful in other types such as allergic and hormonal headaches.

For some patients, magnesium supplementation combined with eliminating food and additive triggers from the diet, results in 100 per cent improvement. The worst offender in this case is the additive MSG (its number on labels will be 621), which is found in many common foods.

For women, there is sometimes a hormonal factor to their headaches. This can be treated with a herbal medicine called Chaste Tree (*Vitex agnus castus*), in combination with zinc and vitamin B6 (usually given in a high-dose B complex). Some women have a better improvement with natural bio-identical progesterone cream instead of Chaste Tree.

For persistent headaches we look further. Mercury from amalgam fillings and low vitamin D levels can again be the problem.

The exciting part of this type of prescribing (apart from the thrill of consistently stretching your intellect) is that the worst result is no improvement.

The best part? No fatalities.

● | THOSE FABULOUS FATTY ACIDS

It is widely known that the high percentage of fat in the diet of Western industrial nations is a major factor in many chronic degenerative illnesses, including cardiovascular disease, diabetes and some cancers.

However, as we said in Chapter 5, not all fats are bad. EFAs, or essential fatty acids, are the basic building blocks in every living cell. They are required for the structure of all cell membranes, giving them flexibility and permeability which are essential to their functioning. They are the precursors in the creation of prostaglandins, which are required for the regulation of almost all body tissues, and they transport and metabolise cholesterol. We do not make EFAs in our bodies so they must be supplied in our food.

Deficiency was commonly seen in babies fed early formulas that lacked essential fatty acids. They tended to develop dry scaly skin, irritability and were prone to respiratory infections.

There are two basic categories of EFAs: omega-3 and omega-6. Omega-3 is found as ALA (alpha-linolenic acid) which is derived from plants: linseed (flaxseed), walnuts and green leafy vegetables, and a much more potent source, EPA (eicosapentaenoic acid) and DHA (docosahexaenoic acid) from fish. Fatty fish such as salmon, herrings, sardines and mackerel are higher in omega-3 than crustaceans (like crab and shrimp) and molluscs (such as mussels, oysters and scallops).

Linoleic acid (LA) is the main omega-6 and is the major EFA in vegetable oils such as sunflower, safflower, soy and corn oil.

Both EFAs are important to us, but our Western diet often has too much omega-6 and insufficient omega-3. This is because the most commonly used oils are high in omega-6 and deficient in omega-3, and many people don't eat enough fish. Research shows that only about 15 per cent of omega-6 is converted to EPA and it may not convert to DHA at all. This conversion is inhibited by a diet high in trans-fatty acids and alcohol and deficient in zinc, vitamins B6 and B3 and magnesium.

Why is this important? Omega-3 easily and quickly converts to anti-inflammatory and anti-pain prostaglandins. Omega-6 may convert but the process is much more complicated, involving many more biochemical pathways; it is therefore much slower and dependent on other nutrients. So to ensure less pain and inflammation in our bodies we need to balance our intake of these EFAs. Specifically, DHA is good for our brains, assisting with learning and behavioural problems; EPA is more beneficial to our hearts.

Research has shown that adding fish to the diet significantly reduces our risk of dying from heart disease and stroke. Epidemiological studies (these look at entire populations) support the idea that fish consumption is inversely related to cardiovascular disease. The more fish eaten, the less heart disease. In some studies this is reduced by 50 per cent, especially if it is fatty fish.

Omega-3s reduce inflammation, so they have a role in treating allergic and inflammatory diseases such as arthritis, inflammatory bowel disease, acne, PMS, eczema, asthma and psoriasis.

The basis of the relationship between fish oils and inflammatory disease comes from observational studies comparing the Inuit people of Greenland and the population of Denmark. Very little inflammatory disease occurs in the Inuit. The biochemistry behind this is linked to AA (arachidonic acid), which is a compound found in meat, shellfish and dairy products. AA forms other compounds in the body that promote inflammation. Eating fish oils has been observed to be associated with a significant reduction in the production of these pro-inflammatory compounds and an increase in anti-inflammatory ones.

Omega-6s do have some proven clinical benefits to health, however. They are known to lower cholesterol levels, and exert positive benefits in cases of eczema, PMS, breast pain, post-natal depression, hypertension and diabetic neuropathy.

The best source of omega-6 is good quality evening primrose oil (EPO). It has anti-inflammatory effects that operate through a different pathway from omega-3, making it useful in milder forms of pain and inflammation. More severe forms usually require omega-3 in high doses initially, after which some conditions can be maintained with EPO.

We recommend that you eat at least as much fish as you do meat, to help keep inflammation in check. Meat provides iron and other minerals but is high in the pro-inflammatory AA; fish counters this effect by reducing inflammation. This is a good reason to eat more fish. It is even better to maintain high levels of dietary omega-3 *and* decrease our intake of high omega-6 saturated fat and edible vegetable oils, as these have the additional downside of interfering with the incorporation of the omega-3s into our body tissues.

It's all about balance — getting the 3:6 ratio right. You may need to see an expert who can make the correct recommendations for you.

Assisting our immune system

One thing we get asked daily at HMC is: 'How do I boost my (or my children's) immune system?'

Modern orthodox medicine battles disease directly by means of drugs, surgery, radiation and other therapies, but many diseases can be avoided — and optimal health attained — by maintaining a healthy, well-functioning immune system. It is the immune system that fights off disease-causing microorganisms and engineers the healing process. In simple terms, the immune system identifies those things that are 'self' and those that are 'foreign'. It then neutralises the 'foreign' things through a system of complex interactions involving the white blood cells, bone marrow, the lymphatic system and serum factors in the blood. I love the image of our white blood cells being soldiers always at the ready to attack invaders.

The immune system needs to be well cared for to work properly. This means getting the right nutrients and avoiding things that depress it. Many elements in our environment compromise the ability of this intricately balanced system. Chemicals, environmental pollutants, stress, the myriad of additives in food, and overuse of antibiotics and other drugs are some of these.

Antibiotics, for instance, only assist with bacterial illnesses but are sometimes given during a viral illness to prevent the development of a bacterial illness. We believe this represents an overuse of these drugs. Another common overuse is the systematic dosing of animals kept at close quarters in feedlots and battery sheds, as described in Chapter 6. The main problem with these overuses is that they cause bacteria to develop resistance to the medications, so the medications don't work when they are really needed. This is becoming a major problem in the Western world.

The following is a list of some important nutrients as well as tips to support healthy immune function. Please note that with these, as with any nutrients, we prescribe based on diagnosed individual needs. We do not endorse random supplementation.

Vitamin C

It is important to maintain a regular intake of vitamin C, because our bodies cannot make it. Eating fresh vegetables and fresh fruit (or fresh fruit and vegetable juices) is therefore essential on a daily basis.

Prolonged stress, infection and trauma burn up vitamin C faster than normal. These conditions produce adrenaline, which in part is made from vitamin C. There are also high concentrations of this vitamin in white blood cells, which are our strong line of defence against illness, so if too much is being used in making adrenaline, more is needed to keep adequate white blood cell numbers. Smoking also causes serious depletion. Alcohol and some medications, like the oral contraceptive pill and steroids, lower the body's vitamin C levels as well.

Vitamin C is a powerful antioxidant. Oxidation is the process where the cells in the body are split or oxidised resulting in highly reactive chemicals called free radicals. These free radicals can damage important cellular molecules such as DNA, lipids or other parts of the cell because they are highly charged, due to having unpaired electrons. This is one of the main processes in the ageing of our cells and bodies. Vitamin C has a powerful anti-ageing effect, neutralising free radical molecules by donating an electron, which stops the free radicals from damaging our cells. Amen to that!

It is also involved in many biological reactions in the body that stimulate growth and repair. It helps with the absorption of iron, the metabolism of connective tissue and the synthesis of some of the body's hormones.

Studies show that vitamin C significantly reduces the symptoms and duration of a number of illnesses. This is because it activates two of the body's white blood cells, the neutrophils and phagocytes, which attack bacteria. Vitamin C also raises levels of interferon, which directly attacks viruses. Finally, there is strong evidence that this remarkable vitamin has a protective effect against cancers.

It is best taken in the form of healthy organic food sources, which naturally contain vitamin C as well as synergistic vitamins, enzymes and coenzymes, trace mineral activators and many other nutrients (both known and unknown). We prescribe it therapeutically in a high-quality, practitioner-only form that includes some of these goodies that come from the food sources, and achieve great results.

Zinc

Zinc is an integral component of many enzyme processes in the body. It synthesises and stabilises proteins, DNA and RNA (cellular genetic protein synthesis materials). It is a structural component of cell membranes and is absolutely required for normal sperm manufacture and the growth and development of embryos and foetuses. Zinc is crucial in decreasing inflammation and reducing the predisposition to inflammation. It plays an important role in the production of white blood cells that fight off illness.

Studies say it is also effective in significantly reducing symptoms of tinnitus, is responsible for optimal functioning of the eye, great for acne and helps with PMS too.

Mild zinc deficiency has been related to many conditions, such as diabetes, alcoholism, inflammatory bowel disease, asthma, low-protein diets, taking the oral contraceptive pill and malabsorption syndromes. A mild deficiency can cause stunted growth in children, decreased taste sensation, impaired immune system and night blindness.

The best dietary source of zinc is oysters. Pine nuts, pecans and other nuts, pumpkin and sunflower seeds, whole grains and most animal proteins are the next best sources, but all contain a lot less zinc than oysters.

We diagnose deficiency with a blood test and supplement as needed. General zinc supplementation can also be beneficial at the beginning of many infections; where appropriate, we prescribe elemental zinc.

Selenium

Selenium serves to protect proteins, cell membranes, lipids and nucleic acids from damaging oxidative molecules. It is vital in the process of converting our thyroid hormone into its active form. Low levels are often reported in people with heart disease and certain cancers. This mineral is especially important if you have amalgam fillings in your teeth (see heavy metal poisoning, page 184).

Tests have shown that New Zealand soils have very low amounts of selenium, meaning that we often get insufficient amounts of it in our diets. Brazil nuts contain high amounts of selenium and you can get enough by eating three a day.

Supplementation starts at 150 µg (in the elemental form) daily for adults and can be great for helping immune function, but we only do this in conjunction with blood test results.

Selenium is used in the body in the form of selenocysteine. Selenomethionine is the most well absorbed form and sodium selenate may also be used in certain situations. Please note that selenium is toxic in doses over 400 µg a day, so it's not something to start swallowing without professional advice.

Vitamin A

Vitamin A also plays many roles in maintaining a healthy immune system and its metabolites are essential for vision and reproduction. Carotenoids (from dark green, orange, yellow and red fruits and vegetables) convert in the bowel to vitamin A. There are more than 600 carotenoids in nature and about 50 of them can be metabolised into vitamin A. Children with vitamin A deficiency have increased incidence of infections, diarrhoea and respiratory illnesses. To get sufficient vitamin A to maintain a healthy immune system, we recommend that people eat plenty of kumara, pumpkin and carrots (three glasses of carrot juice per week is ideal). Eaten in the vegetable form like this there is no risk of hypervitaminosis or toxicity as the betacarotinoids only selectively convert to vitamin A.

However, we sometimes do prescribe it in the form of halibut liver oil or cod liver oil — not exactly yummy, but so beneficial. Luckily it comes in capsules. Too much pure vitamin A can be toxic and high doses are not advisable during pregnancy.

Vitamin D

Vitamin D is made in our bodies when the skin is exposed to sunlight. When exposed to the sun's ultraviolet rays, a cholesterol component in the skin is transformed into a precursor to vitamin D. Active vitamin D is synthesised in the liver. Levels can be measured with a blood test.

Its action in the body is more like a hormone than a vitamin. What's the difference? A hormone is a chemical substance that is secreted into body fluids and transported to an organ or other tissue, where it produces a specific effect on metabolism. Vitamins are organic micronutrients, present in minute quantities in natural foodstuffs, which are essential to normal metabolism.

Vitamin D is needed for the absorption of calcium to create strong bones and teeth and a deficiency will cause muscular aches and pains, sleep problems and depression. It is usually low in diabetics and is important in sugar metabolism. There are many studies using vitamin D in the prevention and treatment of many types of cancer, and we have found that patients who develop cancer often have very low levels. Among those with active cancer it can be very difficult to get vitamin D up to sufficient levels, even with prescription cholecalciferol, which contains 1.25 mg or 50,000 International Units of vitamin D.

Sunlight is known to increase serotonin levels within the body (and therefore melatonin) and vitamin D is widely known as an excellent remedy for both depression and disrupted sleep patterns. One can surmise that vitamin D from the sun that aids the production of serotonin and consequently melatonin, although this has not yet been proven. Many people find that their mood is more flat and sleep quality poor during the winter months. We have found over and over again that when we correct vitamin D levels, our patients experience a dramatic improvement in their quality of sleep and significantly elevated mood. We can deduce that vitamin D improves melatonin and serotonin levels, but we cannot measure these in the body and are therefore unable to prove this.

Exposing the arms and legs to daylight (not necessarily sunshine) for 15 minutes a day can provide enough vitamin D. However, people with darker skin need longer in the sun to produce the same amount. Recent evidence suggests that at high noon in midsummer, a dark-skinned person with 80 per cent of their body uncovered needs 60–80 minutes of sunlight to get their daily dose of vitamin D, whereas a pale-skinned person under the same conditions needs just 3–4 minutes! Darker-skinned people who cover large portions of their body, such as those of Indian descent, often have very low vitamin D levels. Interestingly, in New Zealand the normal range for vitamin D on a blood test is 50–150 μmol/l, but the optimum range (especially for those with diabetes or feelings of low mood) is 100–150. We use prescription vitamin D to boost low levels found on blood testing.

Dietary sources of vitamin D include:

- cod liver oil
- halibut liver oil
- atlantic pickled herring
- mackerel
- salmon
- sardines
- eel.

Boron

Boron is a mineral that is also useful in the metabolism of vitamin D. The dietary sources in order of highest concentration are:

- Tomatoes
- Pears

- Apples
- Prunes
- Raisins.

Herbal remedies

There are two powerful herbal remedies that act well on the immune system, echinacea and astragalus.

Echinacea

Echinacea works by increasing and mobilising the white blood cells called lymphocytes, which target the neutralisation of viruses. It also stimulates other important immune factors called T cells (originally thought to be from the 'thymus gland', hence the 'T') and interferon. Because of this it can be extremely helpful in the initial stages of acute illnesses/infection.

We use a tablet form that contains very close to 50 per cent *Echinacea purpurea* root, 50 per cent *Echinacea angustifolia* root. The best part to use is the root (flowering/aerial parts have a lot less bioactive components). The best species to use are *E. angustifolia* (the strongest) and *E. purpurea* — in a blend as close to 50:50 as you can find. We use practitioner-strength tablets four times daily in acute situations. Each tablet contains 600 mg *E. angustifolia* root and 675 mg *E. purpurea* root from cold percolation. (Cold percolation extraction is preferred because it better maintains the quality of the echinacea.)

Note: People with serious conditions such as HIV should use echinacea or any herbal supplements only under the guidance of a medical advisor. Herbal supplements are medicines and can have complex interactions with other medicines. They are best used under the guidance of a specialist practitioner.

Astragalus

If you are suffering from recurring or chronic infections (longer than six weeks), then astragalus is the best choice of herbal medicine. A blood test is useful at this stage to check that the white blood cell count is in the high–normal range. If it is low, then zinc, selenium and adequate protein will help to increase numbers and thus boost immunity.

Hair allergy tests and immunity

We do a hair allergy test for some people with recurrent infections to isolate which foods and/or additives are a burden to their immune system. Many patients, especially children, find that a temporary elimination of these substances provides a great improvement in their immunity and a disappearance of chronic problems.

Bowel absorption

After any antibiotic therapy or bout of diarrhoea we suggest replacement of the healthy bacteria in the gut with a high quality probiotic. Antibiotics are non-selective in the removal of bacteria from your body, so they will take them all, good and bad, and can leave your body bereft of the healthy bacteria it needs to function. The bacteria in your gut are vitally important as they provide the means to absorb the nutrients in your food effectively. Healthy bowel flora convert carotene to vitamin A, make vitamin K and a host of B vitamins, as well as preventing stomach bugs. It goes like this: think of a full bus . . . there is no room for foreign bugs to sit or stand and no room for existing bugs (e.g. *Candida* species) to excessively proliferate. So the healthy balance is maintained. Only good guys on the bus!

If you experience any bloating, wind or queasiness after antibiotics or a stomach bug then taking a probiotic is essential. A good probiotic should settle these symptoms in about one week. If you have had a tummy bug that does not seem to be resolving itself (especially if you have consumed suspect food or water), then you may need to take *Saccaromyces boulardii* (SB). SB is non-colonising yeast that increases secretory IgA (immune protein) production by the mucosa in the gut. It prevents the adherence of pathogens (bacteria, viruses and protozoa) and has a long history of use in Europe for 'traveller's diarrhoea'.

Regular, enjoyable exercise and stress modification are also important for healthy immune function and if you are not sleeping well this needs to be addressed.

CASE STUDY 15

Last year we had an 11-month-old boy who had taken four courses of antibiotics due to respiratory infections and had developed a wheeze and 'rattly' chest. He had been put on asthma medications two weeks prior to seeing us. Following a hair allergy test we identified a problem with a newly introduced formula. After changing to a different formula he only had minor viral infections and an occasional cough, which we managed homeopathically. His chest remained clear without the asthma medications. He has only needed antibiotics once in the last nine months and he has not been to see us at all for respiratory illness for the last six months.

Inflammatory bowel disease

Inflammatory bowel disease is a debilitating condition that can have serious lifelong complications. It is another ailment that responds well to a nutritional approach. One of our most persevering patients taught us a great deal with his journey.

CASE STUDY 16

A 32-year-old man came to us in 2004 after he had left hospital following a particularly bad flare-up of Crohn's disease (a type of inflammatory bowel disease). He had lost blood, was anaemic, and looked and felt dreadful. He was on a strong dose of steroidal anti-inflammatory medication as well as an immune suppressant, which made him feel awful, and he was continuing to have symptoms. His biggest concern was that he and his wife wanted to have a baby, which he was not able to do on the immune suppressant medication.

We put him onto a soft-food diet, which meant most of his food was cooked, and eliminated the foods that he did not handle well — particularly dairy foods. We also prescribed herbal and nutritional anti-inflammatory supplements. This provided a great improvement for him, but he could not stray at all from the dietary guidelines without creating another flare-up (although to a much lesser degree than previously). We all agreed that this did not provide much quality of life for him or his family.

He persevered, and eventually was able to stop the immune suppressant medication so he could start a family, which was a fantastic milestone. This took a lot of commitment for the best part of a year. However, he was not able to stop the steroid medication, which continued to make him feel dreadful, and he was still having mild to moderate flare-ups whenever he strayed from the dietary guidelines.

After reviewing his entire history and progress we discovered that the original problem had been a gastrointestinal bug that he picked up while on holiday in the Pacific Islands. This had progressed to irritable bowel for some years and eventually became inflammatory bowel. This provided an essential clue for his treatment. We gave him Saccharomyces boulardii (SB), a non-colonising yeast that is very beneficial for 'travellers diarrhoea' and can be used effectively in many gastrointestinal infections. This provided a dramatic improvement — all his bleeding and diarrhoea had ceased within two days. He continued symptom-free for three months, so stopped his steroidal anti-inflammatories.

We gradually weaned him off all supplements over the next two months, and apart from some minor proctitis he felt great and continued to remain symptom-free for 12 months without any pharmaceutical or natural medications.

It's been two years since he started treatment and he and his wife have recently had a beautiful baby. He recently had a minor flare-up, which he quickly got under control in one week with prednisone (a steroidal anti-inflammatory). He had been running his body pretty hard and eating all the wrong things

for a time before the flare-up, but was still very happy with the quality of his health and his quality of life.

Our patient has an astonishing quality of life compared to many people other with this disease; they can continue on a gradual decline until they have portions of their bowel removed or, in some cases, have their whole bowel removed and replaced with a colostomy bag. He's had to make significant improvements to his nutrition and take very good care of himself, but for both him and his wife the results have been magnificent.

Irritable bowel syndrome

Another condition that reacts well to a nutritional approach is irritable bowel syndrome, which is usually diagnosed in the absence of any clinical findings. Generally there is a combination of any or all of the following symptoms: bloating, wind, grumbling and loose bowels, or loose bowels alternating with constipation.

It is important to check for other medical conditions and to blood-test for coeliac disease (a condition where people are highly allergic to gluten, which is a protein in wheat, rye, oats and barley). It is then necessary to establish when the symptoms began. If they started after a stomach bug or a course of antibiotics, probiotics are essential.

CASE STUDY 17

A patient called us recently to thank us for the probiotic prescribed. She had experienced digestive problems ever since having an operation and taking antibiotics several years before. After a few days her symptoms were gone and she felt remarkably better.

If problems did not start in this way, the most important thing is to determine any food intolerances. We use a hair allergy test that includes a long list of foods, additives and environmental irritants. After identifying intolerances, temporary elimination of the foods and additives that tested positive is required. Usually these things can be reintroduced, but with decreased frequency.

CASE STUDY 18

An elderly lady came to us after having bowel surgery two years earlier with the usual post-surgical antibiotic treatment. She had suffered from an irritable bowel with wind and diarrhoea ever since. We gave her probiotics and within a week her symptoms had resolved completely. More than one year later she is still symptom-free.

We believe that it is very important to take probiotics after antibiotics and if you take them during your illness this can prevent the wind, nausea, bloating and thrush that normally develop. Again, the key here is the quality of the supplement. Good probiotics contain billions of live bacteria and need to have been refrigerated properly throughout production and shipping. We consider a supplement that contains *Bifidum* species to be very useful, but new evidence about different useful species is coming out all the time. Basically, the probiotic should stop all digestive symptoms and prevent the thrush that occurs with antibiotic use. If it doesn't, it's not good enough and you should seek professional advice.

● | MYCOPLASMA

As mentioned earlier, some of the work at our practice involves integrating traditional and nutritional medicine. Through research carried out by Dr Ann Kopelson, we have recently become aware of the importance of mycoplasma in certain illnesses and have had great results in treating this via an integrated approach.

Mycoplasma are the smallest known self-replicating life form that infect humans. They are tiny anaerobic bacteria that have no cell wall and live inside the cells of humans and animals. They are parasites in our bodies that scavenge proteins, lipids

In the long run,
population is perhaps
the biggest of all
sustainability issues.
We are currently
outstripping our ability
to regenerate resources
by 125%. By 2050 it
will be 200%.

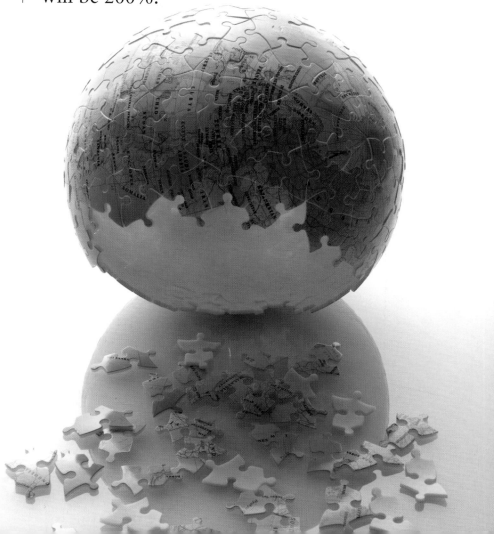

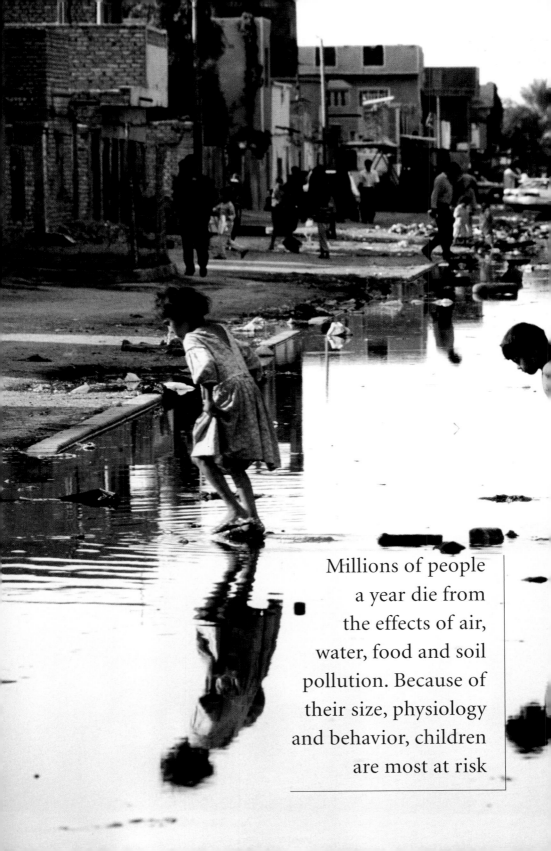

Millions of people
a year die from
the effects of air,
water, food and soil
pollution. Because of
their size, physiology
and behavior, children
are most at risk

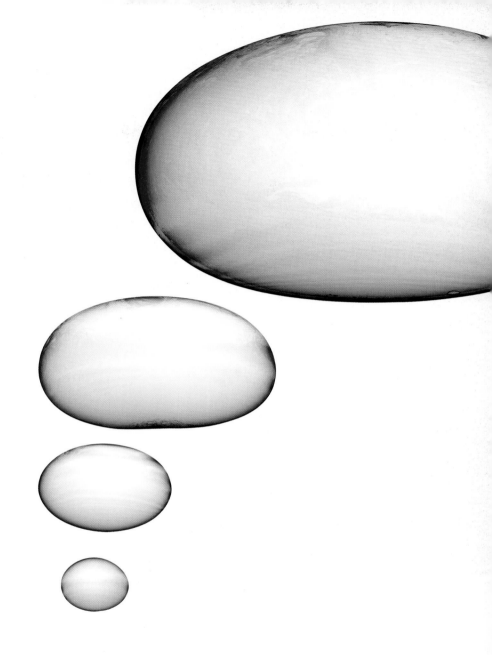

In short, biofuel would seem
to be about the dumbest
solution yet suggested for
our current problems.

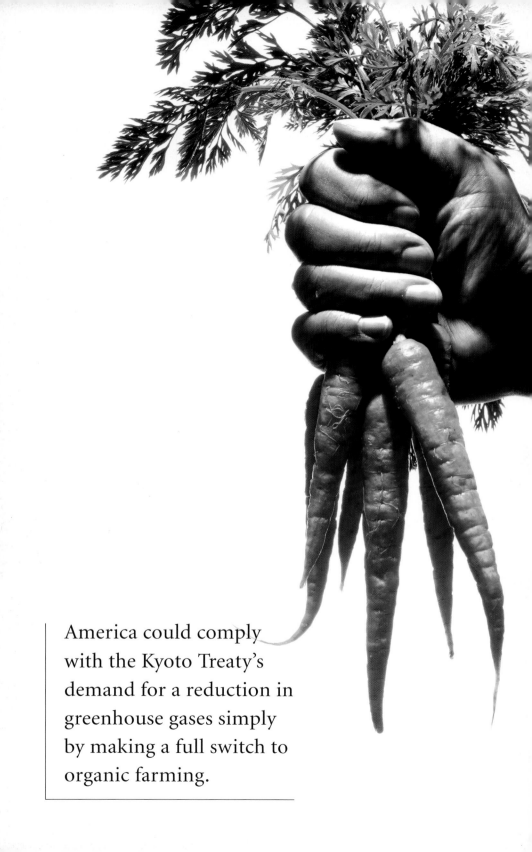

America could comply with the Kyoto Treaty's demand for a reduction in greenhouse gases simply by making a full switch to organic farming.

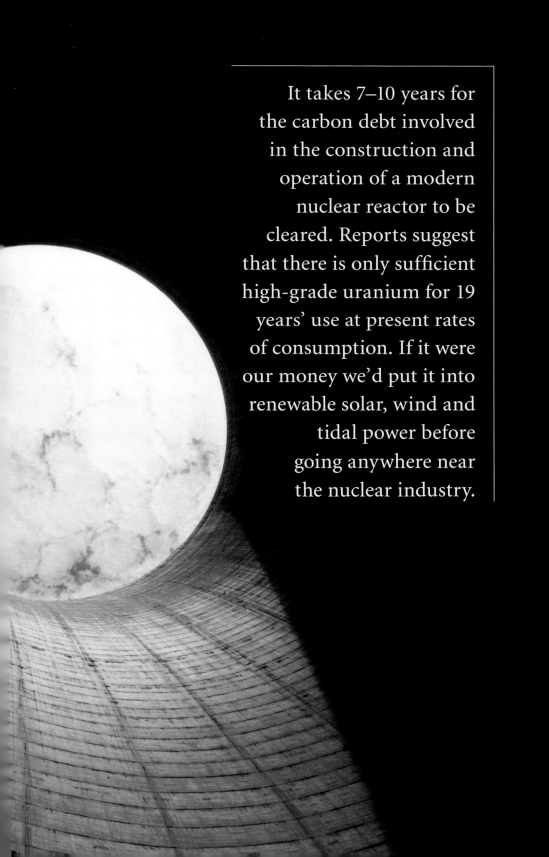

It takes 7–10 years for the carbon debt involved in the construction and operation of a modern nuclear reactor to be cleared. Reports suggest that there is only sufficient high-grade uranium for 19 years' use at present rates of consumption. If it were our money we'd put it into renewable solar, wind and tidal power before going anywhere near the nuclear industry.

Subsidies must be removed and taxes must introduced that reflect the true cost to society of various activities. If this does not occur, Victorian-age technologies will stay in place, blocking the advent of clean, sustainable alternatives that are available right now.

Farm chemicals currently kill up to 67 million birds a year in the US alone.

We're confident that the human race will display its most noble and inspirational traits in rising to, and ultimately overcoming these most dire threats. But it won't be easy, which is all the more reason to get started now.

and sterols to be able to survive and replicate. There are over 70 types of mycoplasma, but only some cause disease. In medical literature there is a strong documented association with heart disease, respiratory illness, arthritis, muscle pain and a host of other conditions. These tiny bacteria thrive in a low-oxygen, acid environment and are sensitive to tetracycline antibiotics.

It is possible to test blood for antibodies to mycoplasma but usually only one type, *Mycoplasma pneumonia*, is available in the testing labs. This organism is associated with pneumonia but it is possible for a patient to have antibodies without having had a respiratory illness.

There is vast information on this topic but we want to share one remarkable case study:

CASE STUDY 19

Several months ago we met a 50-year-old man who had suffered a heart attack three years earlier. Following this he had had three bypass surgeries, replacing the coronary arteries and then replacing stents, which had in turn become blocked as a result of elevated cholesterol. He was unable to take cholesterol-lowering medication due to side effects, so his cholesterol remained elevated.

He presented to us with pain and stiffness all over his body, and marked breathlessness and fatigue. This stopped him from doing any exercise and he could not sleep due to the pain.

When we tested his blood the results were normal, apart from elevated cholesterol and *Mycoplasma pneumonia* antibodies. So we decided to treat him for mycoplasma infection. This treatment involves antibiotics, probiotics, B vitamins to kick start the Krebs (energy) cycle in the body, vitamin C and an alkalising diet to change the environment that mycoplasma thrive in.

> Within six weeks his cholesterol levels were normal, much to the surprise of his cardiologist, and he was experiencing less pain at night.
>
> Two weeks later his only pain was morning stiffness. He had no breathlessness and was back at the gym and walking long distances — a very happy man.
>
> If you would like further information on mycoplasma, contact *annkopelson@yahoo.com*.

Summary

CASE STUDY 20

From a patient's letter: 'You may think we are going elsewhere for medical care but we are not. The guidelines you have given us to maintain our own health must be working too well . . . we have been very healthy. I am so grateful to all, because you took so much time to be thorough in your diagnosis . . . so much time and most important of all, you got it right! Your natural therapies have worked out cheaper — 1) because THEY WORKED, 2) because we have learnt some ways to prevent further problems, and 3) because repeat visits have proved unnecessary.'

For the doctors working in this way at HMC, seeing patients become really well provides a huge sense of satisfaction and joy. The depth of research, peer discussion and support we experience affirms our confidence in the continued development of this approach to medicine. We dream that one day every doctor will learn and practise nutritional medicine alongside pharmacology (the prescribing of drugs); that the food menus in hospitals will change to become truly healthy and so aid healing; and that we as doctors will radiate superb health as an inspiration to our patients! The Hippocratic Oath that we all sign as we graduate states: 'Do no harm.' Hippocrates also said, 'Let thy food be thy medicine and thy medicine be thy food.' These are the values that we live and practise medicine by.

It may sound simplistic, but we see our bodies as being like gardens. Most of us reap what we sow. For sure, there are lots of people who suffer from random illnesses that strike without reason, but many diseases are preventable and are more easily treated when we take the time and care to feed and nourish our bodies with high-quality nutrients. Eating whole foods, grown organically, is the best place to start, and with careful diagnosis and individual prescription it's possible to combine traditional medical thinking with nutritional medicine to ensure that you live your most vital life. **)**

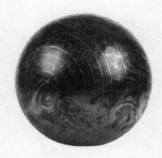

part three|global energy

If we can successfully face the ecological challenges of the next 50 years, Planet Earth could be a pretty cool place to live in the future. Governments, businesses and individuals all have a part to play and *you* can make a difference.

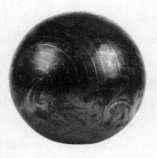

8 | global weirding

We're writing this after abandoning a planned post-conference ski trip to the Alps, owing to a lack of snow. The Swiss and Austrian tourist industries are talking disaster in the wake of their warmest early winter on record. At the same time the media is full of comment about the Stern Report on the punitive costs of failing to address climate change (see Introduction).

Against this backdrop, there are still those who suggest that the projected rise in temperatures of three to four degrees Celsius this century is not a big deal and others who argue that tackling greenhouse gases will impose unnecessary costs. For anyone trying to make sense of all the controversy there's a more worrying question: if the experts are right, what possible difference can my own household make? Over the next few pages we hope to give you enough facts to make an informed judgment on the issue, and in Chapter 13 we make suggestions for simple steps you can take immediately if you're keen to be part of the solution.

The first thing worth thinking about is some of the labels given to the various bits of the puzzle. The Irish physicist John Tyndall first suggested the idea of the greenhouse effect in 1863, when people in his part of the world were a lot more familiar with greenhouses. If he was naming it today he would probably call it the 'parked car on a summer's day' effect and most of us would have an instant grasp of what it's all about. We'd understand that the consequences of this effect are pretty unpleasant, whereas greenhouses conjure up images of productivity and luscious fruit and flowers. The glass windows let the sun's energy in and then trap it inside the car in exactly the same way that gases in the atmosphere trap some of the sun's energy on Earth. More gases equal thicker windows. Doubling the concentration of gases, which the world is in the process of doing, means we might as well be double-glazing the car.

Global warming is another term with a benign ring to it, suggesting that we should all lie around while things warm up a bit. People in colder climates joke about needing more sun. The eminent English scientist who developed the Gaia theory of the Earth as a living system, James Lovelock, also dislikes the term global warming because 'it is too cosy'. He prefers 'global heating' because it has a starkness about it. 'Climate change' is a more accurate expression and also encompasses the devastation caused by Hurricane Katrina in 2005 and sister storms, but it is still a dispassionate term. A more descriptive title for the weather ahead of us was coined by the American energy guru Amory Lovins: 'global weirding'. Somehow, global weirding captures the situation when we have extreme cold snaps while there is an overall warming trend, and covers the really major climate events that are going on around the world, such as droughts that last for decades in Australia.

The greenhouse gas we hear the most about is carbon dioxide (CO_2). This is the stuff that we breathe out and living plants give off at night. It makes up a puny 0.0383 per cent of the Earth's atmosphere compared to the heavyweight non-greenhouse gases — nitrogen (78.084 per cent) and oxygen (20.946 per cent). Another major greenhouse gas is methane, which accounts for an even more minuscule 0.000175 per cent. Methane is a problem because each molecule has the insulating or greenhouse power of 23 CO_2 molecules. Methane comes from any organic matter that rots in the absence of air (anaerobically) as well as from the burping of grazing animals. This is important for New Zealanders because a few years ago the Government tried to introduce a carbon tax that was going to include emissions from the agricultural sector. The Opposition promptly relabelled this a 'fart tax'. It didn't matter that they were anatomically mistaken. The label stuck and the Government had to drop the whole idea, although it was quite a good one and will doubtless resurface in the future.

The big issue with methane is the enormous quantities of vegetation buried in the permafrost of Siberia. It has not decomposed since being frozen solid during the last Ice Age. Even a slight amount of warming makes more of this material available to rot, resulting in a rapid escalation in the amount of methane in the atmosphere. This situation is called a positive feedback loop, where the cycle takes over and becomes the major, and ongoing, source of greenhouse gases.

Water vapour is another contributory factor. Its concentration in the atmosphere varies between one and four per cent. Increased warming means there will be more of it in the atmosphere, which adds another feedback loop and another potential tipping point.

An element of doubt?

Looking a bit more closely at these figures we learn that the 0.0383 per cent share of the atmosphere that is CO_2 represents 383 individual CO_2 molecules for every million molecules measured by volume. Before we started the wholesale use of fossil fuels, beginning with coal to power the Industrial Revolution in the 18th and 19th centuries, the level of CO_2 in the atmosphere was 280 parts per million. Since then it's increased to 383 parts per million and is on track to reach double the pre-Industrial Revolution concentration in the near future.

The only question that has ever been in doubt is whether or not the quantities of fossil fuels (oil, coal, natural gas etc) that people are using worldwide are sufficient to have an effect on the climate, or whether the extra CO_2 might be coming from elsewhere. Here are a few points that might help you answer that question:

1. There is no one who denies the existence of a greenhouse effect, where the atmosphere traps some incoming solar radiation. Without it the

Earth would be permanently freezing — similar to Venus and quite unsuited to life.

2. Atmospheric concentration of greenhouse gases has dramatically increased over the last 200 years. Antarctic ice-core studies show that CO_2 concentration during this period has increased by around 40 per cent on its level for the prior 10,000 years, with *half* of that increase occurring in the last 35 years. Methane has increased by 150 per cent!

3. The fourth report of the Intergovernmental Panel on Climate Change (IPCC) issued in early 2007 was quite clear: there was a 90 per cent chance that human industrial activity had caused changes in climate and the situation was set to get much worse. If you want to test that, try the common sense model again.

If you look at a map of the central North Island you'll find Lake Taupo, which was formed in a massive volcanic eruption some 26,000 years ago. Lake Taupo's most recent eruption was in AD 186 and geologists tell us it was the largest volcanic event on Earth in the last 5000 years. Sixty-five million tonnes of rock, dust and gases were ejected into the atmosphere. Scholars in China and Rome recorded the effect of this eruption, noting red skies at sunrise and sunset and a general lack of brightness from the sun.

By comparison, we are currently using 4629 million tonnes of hard coal and 3847 million tonnes of oil annually, and putting their combustion products into the atmosphere. That's 8467 million tonnes compared with 65 million tonnes when Lake Taupo erupted. Absolutely staggering. We're talking about 130 times the impact! The Taupo eruptions caused visible climate change for a few years; to expect no impact to our climate from doing something similar 130 times every year, year after year, would appear just a little optimistic.

Sequestration

We have been mining fossil fuels at a colossal rate, extracting material created over millions of years and using it within a few human generations. Common sense says we cannot do this with impunity unless there is somewhere that the excess carbon can go as a part of natural cycles. The fact that we are seeing steadily rising CO_2 levels in the atmosphere suggests that there are insufficient natural sinks into which it is being poured.

However, carbon *can* be removed from the atmosphere by being absorbed into growing trees and that is why we are hearing so much more about tree planting. But we have to be careful about where the trees are planted and about their ultimate fate. Unfortunately, any tree likely to wind up as paper destined for a landfill where it will decompose anaerobically and give off methane will only make matters worse in the long term.

Trees in tropical forests are more effective carbon sinks. While deforestation rates are slowing, the UN's Food and Agriculture Organisation (FAO) reports that we are still annually felling an area the size of Greece. The land is being used to fulfill First World demand for things like tropical hardwoods, beef, soy for animal feed and 'alternative' fuels.

It's essential that we support rainforest protection and permanent reafforestation projects, and lobby our governments to do the same. It's no use saying that it's the problem of the Third World countries concerned. Industrialised countries have created the bulk of the existing problem and we can afford to fix it — they can't.

There may be other cost-effective ways of locking up carbon, called sequestering it, but none is readily apparent. Most methods, such as burying it in disused mine shafts or oil wells, require vast quantities of energy for transportation, and don't consider the consequences of catastrophic failure in an earthquake. We cannot talk of clean coal until the technology is tried and proven, which is currently a long, long way off. While we can keep our fingers crossed for breakthroughs in sequestration technology, we need sustained research and commitment to policies that provide increasing support to non-carbon alternatives into the future.

Kicking the carbon habit

One analogy for the challenge ahead is our fight against smoking. In our parents' era even athletes smoked, and scorn was directed at those who suggested it was harmful. At the peak of its popularity about half of the adult population were smokers, whereas the figure has fallen to just a quarter now. The reduction follows public health campaigns, bans on advertising tobacco products, restrictions on smoking in public places, and punitive (and escalating) taxes.

However, if we halved our present emissions of greenhouse gases, we would still need to halve the remaining production to achieve the estimated 70–80 per cent reduction that is needed to stabilise the climate. We can safely guess that we are going to need something a lot more effective than the measures employed to cut smoking, because we get many more obvious benefits from fossil-fuel energy use and other greenhouse-effect creating activities than are provided by smoking. There will be more pain before we see the gain.

Replacing fossil-fuel energy plays such an important part in beating global warming that we deal with it separately in the following chapter. For a summary of other practical ways in which you can help to solve the problem, see Chapter 13.

To end on a positive note, over the past year we've undergone a dramatic improvement in our expectations about the outcome of this problem. The world seems finally to have focused on the issue and that is an awesome thing to see. Businesspeople and philanthropists are creating new solutions every day. The New Zealand Prime Minister, Helen Clark, has indicated that she wants to see our country lead the way by becoming carbon neutral by 2050. Many other national and local government leaders have stated similar goals. We should not minimise the challenges that this will present but nor should we shrink from the task.

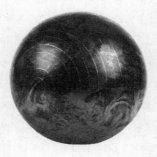

9 | **taming the dragon**

Many of the characteristics that make us human are tied up with energy. We wear clothes and live in shelters in part to conserve it. So many features of the way we live involve harnessing the energy of other creatures and of the earth's natural resources. What other animals light up their worlds and cause so much visual pollution that city dwellers may never see stars in the night sky?

Our ancestors started controlling fire around 500,000 years ago and entered us into a new league — one of both opportunity and destruction.

For probably longer than that, however, humans took advantage of another timeless source of external energy — *other humans* — in many cases, slaves, to improve their production processes and their quality of life.

A physicist at Wellington's Victoria University, Dr Peter Johnston, calculated that the average New Zealander was using the energy equivalent of 300 slaves working for them for 24 hours a day. The total for the average American is closer to 500 slaves.

For all its faults, technology has brought a better life to most of mankind. However, old technologies unintentionally produce pollution that endangers us. And as the number of people using dated technologies has grown exponentially, so too has the danger. We now need to implement new ways of harnessing the earth's resources and in the meantime we have to learn to reduce the amount of 'external' energy we use.

Another Kiwi, Al Forbes, has given us his insight into people and energy by designing and making a low-speed electricity generator powered by pedalling a stationary bike. From his book *The Homebuilt Dynamo* we learn that an hour's vigorous pedalling in the morning generates enough electricity to keep eight 13 watt fluorescent lights working in the evening. The three billion of us worldwide who have electricity would not have enough pedaling hours in the day to keep all the modern appliances in our homes plugged in. The other half of humanity, with no access to electricity, might leap at the prospect of a few hours' pedalling to get the joy of some good, safe lighting or to power the radio. One thing is certain: neither group would pedal to keep the television on standby, using electricity and doing nothing.

Boys from the blackstuff

The use of human, largely slave, labour as well as animal energy started to be replaced by water wheels around AD 500. By AD 1068 there were 6000 water wheels in England and 20,000 in France. At roughly the same time, in Persia, vertical axis windmills were developed. Like water wheels, these were used for grinding grain and pumping water. The first recorded accounts of horizontal axis windmills of the type that we are familiar with can be found in England in AD 1219 and China in AD 1270.

Throughout history, humans have burned wood, peat and dung for cooking and heating, and supplemented this with coal in locations where it washed up from naturally exposed seams. However, in AD 1229 King Henry III of

England granted the first charter to Newcastle-upon-Tyne to dig for coal. This enabled us to enter the era of mega-air-polluters. (The direct result of this was that by the early 1800s the average life expectancy in Nottingham, England, was 19 years.) In AD 1000, the Hopi Indians, in what is now Arizona, were using coal to fire their pottery.

We have already looked at feedback loops and tipping points in relation to climate change, but we can also see them in the history of energy use and the broader Industrial Revolution. The steam engine developed by Newcomen in 1712 was designed to pump water out of mines, allowing more coal to be mined. It had an energy efficiency of 0.5 per cent — roughly one hundredth of the efficiency of a modern diesel engine. Later developments by James Watt turned the steam engine into a railway engine and opened the possibility of moving vast quantities of coal over long distances. At about the same time, in 1748, the first recorded commercial coal production was taking place in America, in the Manakin, Virginia, area. In 1839 the steam shovel was invented, allowing even more prodigious quantities of coal to be removed.

In 1901 the General Electric Company built the first coal-fired alternating current power plant for the Webster Coal and Coke Company of Ehrenfeld, Pennsylvania, and started the wholesale use of coal as a fuel for generating power. By 1961 coal became the main fuel for electricity generation in the US and it remains the number one fuel for power generation worldwide. In 1990, the American coal industry extracted one billion tons of coal for the first time.

In 2000, the US had coal reserves of 246 billion tons. Running out is not a likely prospect in the near future. Many other countries, including New Zealand and China, also have massive reserves of coal, so the prospect of 'peak coal' is not going to arise any time soon. This will pose some very real problems for future decision-makers. We'll get on to that once we've had a look at the current really big player in the energy stakes — oil.

Black gold, Texas tea . . .

It's hard to believe that humanity did not find a use for oil throughout eons of our history before turning it into the cornerstone of our society. The first oil well was drilled by Edwin L Drake in Titusville, Pennsylvania in 1859 at a time when whaling fleets were supplying much of the world with whale oil for lighting. The first oil was refined to make high-grade products to be incorporated into cosmetics, with the bulk cast aside as waste, but very quickly its versatility became apparent.

In 1900 world oil extraction was 20,220,000 metric tons, doubling to 44,212,000 tons in 1910 and doubling again to 94,252,000 tons in 1920. It doubled again to 199,957,000 tons in 1930 and then increased by 50 percent to 302,000,000 tons by 1940. By 1954 it had more than doubled again to 708,740,000 tons and by 1994 it had increased more than four and a half times to 3,318,000,000 tons. In 2004 the total was 3,847,167,000 tons. Nearly four billion tons of sticky black goo is taken out of holes in the ground each year. Add that to coal and natural gas extraction figures and you will find that each year we are taking, in round figures, six billion tons — or one ton of fossil fuel for every human on the planet. And only half of the Earth's people are getting direct benefit.

The only item that we consume in greater quantities is the aggregate that is quarried to make our cities and roads — seven tons per person per year in New Zealand. Obviously, quarrying and rock crushing require vast amounts of energy themselves and the amount of aggregate used to support our modern lifestyles is unbelievable. According to the Aggregate and Quarrying Association of New Zealand, one km of new six-lane highway requires 20,000 tons of crushed aggregate. Small wonder that half of all the energy used in the world today is devoted to the construction sector. However, it is now possible to design buildings that use far less energy in construction and which then reward the occupants with lower energy bills for the rest of their lives — all for the same cost or slightly above.

Peak oil

Talk to anyone about energy and the question of when the oil is going to run out will pop up very quickly. Here's the answer: nobody knows. The countries with the most oil are the ones with the least transparent public records. Based on best guesses, *The Economist* reckons we've got 40 years of oil left at present rates of consumption.

There's a popular idea that the oil will run out, we'll all see the error of our ways, and we'll somehow reform and return to a more benign existence. This seems very unlikely. Yes, the oil will run out, but long before that time our present over-consuming society would have moved to other energy sources, including coal. (That's exactly what we did in World War 2. Cars drove around fuelled by bags of coal gas stored on their roofs.) We are not going to run out of coal in New Zealand for hundreds of years, nor will America or China.

But turning to coal would be a greenhouse gas disaster, because it has many more molecules of carbon for each unit of energy available than oil or natural gas. We need to make the right choices now and not wait for our hands to be forced by resource depletion. This requires our political decision-makers, worldwide, to be much more forward thinking than they have been in the past. We need to *demand* this of them, rather than blundering into the future hoping that we are going to strike it lucky.

Nuclear power

There's something wonderfully human about solving one issue and, in the process, creating other problems with even greater legacies. Nothing fits into this category more clearly than nuclear power, which has received a new lease of life because of its apparently low carbon footprint. The reality is very different, as we will see.

In the heyday of the promotion of nuclear power in the 1960s we were told that the new power plants were going to generate such cheap electricity that the utility companies would not bother to meter or charge for it. That never came to pass.

Nuclear power is, by its nature, very risky. The probability of a serious incident occurring at any given time is very low, but the consequences are potentially devastating — both at the time of the event and thousands of years into the future. Let's take a quick look at the risks and apply the same common sense formula we've used elsewhere.

If any business applied for permission to construct a widget factory and one aspect of making widgets involved the production of a highly hazardous waste that remained toxic for thousands of years, it would be reasonable to expect the company to have a waste disposal plan. For the most part, the nuclear industry has not properly addressed the question of waste and there are well-documented cases of large quantities of radioactive waste being stored in inadequate facilities in the US, England and the former USSR. Before there is any further consideration of nuclear power the waste issue has to be resolved.

In capitalist economies, a new business has to satisfy all its backers and shareholders that it has an adequate business plan, including insurance cover for any eventuality. The nuclear industry needs to meet these same criteria and not turn to governments to cover the extreme risks associated with potential catastrophic damage.

The next major risk associated with the nuclear industry is impossible to quantify because it is associated with security and terrorism. The probability of a terrorist incident at any given nuclear facility may be low, but the consequences if one does occur are potentially huge.

The ostensible reason for a resurgence of interest in nuclear power is its apparently low emissions of greenhouse gases. This may be the case within the actual reactions generating the power, but is by no means true overall. There are two issues. Firstly, the quantity of fossil fuels used in building a nuclear power plant is very large, because they are massive concrete structures and the manufacture of concrete is extremely fossil-fuel greedy. The cartage of tonnes of aggregate would involve vehicles fuelled by fossil fuels, which are also essential in mining, milling, enriching and delivering the uranium fuel.

The Australian scientist Mark Diesendorf has reviewed the literature in this field and suggests it would take between seven and ten years before the carbon debt involved in the construction and operation of a modern reactor could be cleared. Writing in *Australian Science* in July 2005 he further points out that the world has very limited supplies of high-grade uranium, with some reports suggesting there is sufficient for only 19 years' use at present rates of consumption — enough to generate the entire world's electricity for a modest 6.8 years. These figures for the size of the resource do not stack up against the enormous reserves of coal worldwide, which is the predominant source of electricity generation at the moment. After using the high-grade ore, the nuclear industry will have to use lower-grade fuel and this will require vastly more fossil fuel to get it ready to use. At this point nuclear power stations would not beat natural gas in terms of their greenhouse gas profile.

There are other nuclear technologies in the wings that may avoid this greenhouse gas trap, but they are not operational at present and all require vast quantities of government backing to advance beyond the experimental stage. If it were our money we would choose to put it into renewable solar, wind and tidal power before going anywhere near the nuclear industry. We believe that all safe options must be exhausted before nuclear technology comes into the picture.

Biofuels

Another way of approaching the energy issue is to look seriously at biofuels, or ethanol and vegetable oils, as they have in Brazil for many years. This initially appears sensible from the greenhouse gas point of view, because the gases emitted when the fuel is burned will effectively be reabsorbed the following season when a new crop is grown, leaving no net increase in atmospheric loading. It also sounds great in terms of getting rid of waste products such as vegetable oils from restaurants. But the prospect of a wholesale conversion to biofuels just won't work.

Advocating a major shift to biofuels, as President Bush did in his 2007 State of the Union address, would make the US less dependent on imported oil from the Middle East but would condemn many people to effective starvation in the Third World as the price of their staple foodstuffs increased beyond reach. Corn and soy prices have already begun to increase dramatically on world commodities exchanges as a result of competition from the biofuels industry, which in turn creates more competition for other food crops and pushes their prices up as well — the supply and demand forces of the market rule. The only saving grace here for the world's two billion poorest people, who spend up to half their income on food, is that biofuel production becomes uneconomic when prices for the raw materials involved reach the levels that they are already approaching.

Even if we didn't care about the welfare of the world's poorest and could develop less expensive biofuel conversion technologies, American researchers have noted that 'dedicating all present US corn and soybean production to biofuels would meet only 12 per cent of our gasoline demand and six per cent of diesel demand. Total US cropland reaches 625,000 square miles. To replace US oil consumption with biofuels we would need 1.4 million square miles of corn for ethanol and 8.8 million square miles of soybean for biodiesel.' If there were significantly more arable land available in the world without destroying precious forests and grasslands (and there is not), where would the water come from to irrigate any dramatic increase in crop production? Chapter 12 gives an overview of the world's growing water shortage.

Biofuel can also be produced from waste products such as vegetable oils, tallow and (possibly at some time in the future) wood chips. However, forecasts suggest that those materials will soon be in such high demand relative to supply that processors will quickly turn to rainforest-competitive sources such as palm oil and sugar cane.

Finally, it has been estimated that the biofuel industry leads to an actual *increase* in greenhouse gas loading. A 2006 study by researchers at the University of Minnesota pointed out that biofuel crops have to be irrigated, ploughed and harvested, fertilised, transported and distilled using energy intensive processes that ultimately cause a net increase in emissions, to say nothing of their other ecologically undesirable effects.

In short, biofuel substitution would seem to be about the dumbest solution yet suggested for our current problem.

Some smart alternatives

When New Zealand won the America's Cup in 1995, someone said that having used the wind to win the world's oldest international sporting trophy, we should go on and lead the world in the wind power stakes. This was not to be; the Danes probably hold that title for now, with more people employed in the renewable energy field than in their substantial commercial fishing industry.

In the past, New Zealand has been a world leader in terms of expertise in hydro and geothermal power generation. Dams were built on every major river in the first half of last century, much like the US, and we then went on to generate power from naturally occurring volcanic activity in the centre of the North Island. Naturally enough, mistakes were made. Some of the hydro lakes are silting up and the take from some geothermal fields has had to be reduced, but by and large we're blessed with a substantial renewable resource for power generation, providing an enviable 73 per cent of the electricity used in our country in the last quarter of 2004.

There are no single quick-fix solutions to keep up this record and provide ongoing security of supply. There are no major untapped rivers or geothermal fields. Our various power suppliers are going all-out to tap the abundant wind resource with large wind farms, and the prospect of wave power remains tantalising but not ready to switch on. There are, however, a few other smart options.

One promising idea is to combine various existing power saving and generating technologies with the internet era, to give us distributed generation and power grids that work both ways — supplying power and receiving it from small generators when they are not at peak load. Let's take a brief step back and explain how some of the power sources and technologies might be linked in the future.

Like so many technologies on the green agenda, the components have been around for over a century and we are only now realising their practical applications. The Reverend Dr Robert Stirling and his brother James, an engineer, invented the Stirling engine in 1816. They were trying to develop a safer version of the steam engine, which had a habit of exploding in the early days. The Stirling model is an external combustion engine. It's ideal for generating electricity, hot water and heat for households in colder climates from the same input of energy. These engines are very quiet but slow to start up, which is why they lost out to the internal combustion engine used in most motors (except in submarines).

Beginning in 1987, a research team at Canterbury University in Christchurch took the concept of the Stirling engine and combined it with modern combustion and control systems to develop home-scale, gas-fired AC electricity generators, which also provide hot water and heat for homes. This invention was marketed under the WhisperGen brand in 1995, and between 2002 and 2004 was trialled in homes in the UK, with the result that a major British supplier has placed an order for 80,000 units to be installed by 2009. Commercial arrangements for supply of the same units in Europe are being finalised and DC units for remote rural settings are also available. These units are powered by natural gas at the moment but the engines are well-suited to hydrogen fuel, raising the possibility of gradually moving out of the fossil fuel economy.

The same engines are also suited to cooling cycles and can be expected to play a very important role in those large chunks of the world where air conditioning is more of an issue than space heating. To learn more, visit *www. whispergen.com*.

Furthermore, Stirling engines are ideally suited to large applications where massive amounts of heat are required. In 2005, Southern California Edison announced that it was purchasing 20,000 units from a different supplier over 20 years to generate 500 megawatts of electricity from solar power, where the sun's rays are concentrated by a series of specially positioned mirrors on a 19 sq km site.

If Stirling engines seem like a gift from the distant past, then look at the fuel cell. In 1843, Welsh physicist Sir William Grove developed the first working fuel cell from a concept developed by Christian Friedrich Schönbein in 1838–9. Schönbein, a German-Swiss chemist, was also the first to discover ozone, but it is his work on the fuel cell that captivates us now. These gadgets generate electricity by combining hydrogen and oxygen to produce water as a waste product. They were developed further by Americans in the 1950s and 1960s for the space program, and have been refined in various state-supported research programs in Japan since the 1980s. They are now undergoing a large scale trial in Japanese households, powered by hydrogen from LPG or, shortly, from kerosene. Each household has an appliance the size of a filing cabinet alongside the entranceway and it provides for their requirements for hot water and electricity.

These developments raise the serious possibility of a hydrogen economy, possibly replacing natural gas where it is reticulated at present with hydrogen. George Monbiot, author of *Heat*, considers that a reticulated hydrogen system is a possibility for Britain with the hydrogen generated from gasification of coal, with the resulting CO_2 buried.

The mix will vary in different settings, but the great news is that we can now envisage a network that feeds electricity back to the grid if there is a local oversupply or draws it down when required. At a local level, in different communities there might be a mix of solar cells, wind turbines, fuel cells or Stirling engines feeding or drawing from the grid. This is one of those technologies that is difficult to wrap your head around when it's explained on paper, but that's easy to adapt to.

Plugging into the sun

One of the major technologies to fit into the above network will be the fast-evolving field of solar energy. With an unlimited supply of raw material, solar power technology is undoubtedly a major part our future. It divides primarily into two components, each with an important contribution to make: solar water heating and solar voltaics or solar power. Some people have also designed houses to take advantage of the sun for direct heating and passive solar ventilation, and this area of building design is growing.

Solar water heating uses simple technology that has been around for a long time. Water heating accounts for around 40 per cent of the average domestic power bill. Depending on local sunshine hours it's possible to save up to 75 per cent of this and repay installation costs over 10–12 years at today's electricity prices (more quickly if they increase). In 2006 the New Zealand Green Party won a major concession from the Government as a part of the post-election co-operation agreement, in which it agreed to fund the promotion of every aspect of solar water heating and get these simple devices installed in far more than the two per cent of houses presently fitted. The package includes education and promotional components as well as training for installers. Like home insulation, this initiative will pay dividends for years to come and — it's hoped — encourage other developments. The challenge, of course, is for those who can afford it to step up and show the way.

Solar voltaics is a different story. If combined with an alternative source for cooking and solar hot water heating, as well as energy efficient appliances and fittings, it is quite possible to lead a modern life using only solar panels and a bank of batteries. It's more convenient, however, to be able to draw power from the grid when you need it, and sell it back when you're producing more than you need. One Aucklander we know disconnected himself from the grid in 1994 and has only reconnected at his new house so he can feed excess power to the grid. As he points out, while it's cost him $30,000 for the panels on his roof, some people spend that changing their car frequently or buying a few expensive accessories — and he is actually earning a return on his investment.

Developments in this area are moving very rapidly. The state of California has introduced a US$3.2 billion rebate scheme in which people can be reimbursed for around a third of the costs of solarising their homes or businesses. Projections are that the economies created as people switch to solar will be such that they won't have to be subsidised long term. The costs of producing the equipment required will come down as more units are ordered.

phillip ' When I judged the Ernst & Young 2006 World Entrepreneur of The Year competition, one of the top-rated contestants was the German firm Q-cells AG. One of Europe's fastest-growing companies, they are developing solar voltaic design so quickly that they believe it will be cost-competitive with grid power as early as 2009. '

The best solutions are often the simplest

While far better in the long term than building more coal-fired power plants, even the greenest energy sources involve some carbon cost in construction. The most eco-friendly force we have at our fingertips is simple conservation. There are technological advances being made in this area every day, from hybrid cars to energy-efficient lighting and appliances, and computer screens that use a fraction of the electricity of their predecessors. When making our next purchase in any of these areas, it's essential to think about energy efficiency. But in the meantime, we can make a contribution to the planet's health and save ourselves money through simple actions like turning off unused lights and appliances. It's great to buy a low-energy screen, but according to Meridian Energy, the equivalent of seven nuclear power stations are in constant use in the US just to power computers that are left on without being used. We talk in detail about some of the things you can do to conserve energy in Chapter 13.

Finally, let's go back to slaves. Abraham Lincoln and the others who abolished slavery in the US did not suggest cuts of ten per cent in slave numbers or stabilising the figures at 1790 levels. They did not propose an elaborate trading system where you could own slaves if you paid for someone else's slaves to be freed. They clearly identified that the use of slaves as a valid source of external energy had run its course and could no longer be justified. We are in similar situation right now: there are better ways of powering our lives than burning fossil fuels and we need to adopt them as fast as possible.

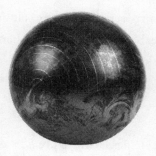

10 | waste not, want not

We're strange creatures. At 0550 GMT on 3 July 2005, NASA achieved the most distant creation of waste possible by directing a washing-machine-sized copper projectile at a comet named Tempel 1, with a closing velocity of 37,100 km per hour; it blasted a hole the size of a football field seven stories deep. All of this took place some 134 million km from Earth. The operation, launched from the Deep Impact spacecraft, cost US$333 million and was aimed at determining the nature of the early solar system.

Psychologists call this sort of behavior displacement; when there are lots of critical things we should be doing, we find one that is far from essential, but possibly interesting, and focus on that. Rather than creating waste in space it might be more useful to look at the mess we're making at home.

Waste has been around a lot longer than human beings. Asteroids, continental drift, ice ages and volcanoes have been producing it in massive quantities for all of history. They've altered the face of continents, flattening certain areas while leaving others intact. Over geological time this physical activity has provided the basis for complex life forms; in turn, the waste products of the biological world have combined with weathered rock to create topsoil, that magical little layer that feeds us all.

These timeless physical and biological processes are natural. They have happened as long as the Earth and its living inhabitants have been around. The difference today is that human intervention has greatly changed the production of these former 'natural' wastes and added some new and frightening compounds to the mix. These observations might appear esoteric, but they have a practical purpose: a big-picture solution to our problems with waste must deal with more than just those that are handled by the local council or driven around in a truck.

A waste of space

The biggest environmental issues facing us are *all* waste issues, although most people will not immediately recognise them as such. Climate change is a waste issue caused by the build-up of waste carbon dioxide and waste methane in the atmosphere, thereby trapping more of the sun's heat. If we reach the tipping point where permafrost starts to melt on a large scale, it will be waste that has made the difference.

The ozone hole was a waste issue. CFCs that escaped from fridges and air conditioners, and those that had been used to make expanded polystyrene, destroyed ozone molecules in the upper atmosphere, leaving a massive hole in the ozone layer that returns each year above Antarctica.

Even the most highly trained technical specialist has difficulty in crediting that waste gases, which we cannot see, weigh enough to worry about. New Zealand produces about four million tons of traditional waste that goes to landfills each year, but according to Environment Ministry figures it also produces 16,712,000 tons of waste gas per annum. Every local authority in New Zealand is required by law to prepare a waste management plan for their area, but none gives more than passing mention to gaseous wastes. We'll discuss possible solutions to this a bit later.

We don't worry about gaseous wastes because we can't see them, but at the other end of the spectrum there are some massive wastes that we can certainly see. New Zealand has some of the most beautiful scenery in the world, with dramatic landscapes that unfold quickly as you explore the country. In March 1988 Cyclone Bola lashed east coast regions of the North Island with torrential rain and hurricane-force winds. It damaged seaside communities and disrupted people's lives, causing erosion of the hillsides on an unprecedented scale. In the years since Bola, the masters of coastal ships heading north have known when to turn left towards Auckland, because the discharge of brown silt from Eastland rivers into the sea has been so great.

Compared to our four million tons of traditional solid waste, the country loses a staggering 400 million tons of sediment from the land to the ocean in an average year — one hundred times as much waste as the traditional rubbish that we take to the dump. This sediment includes an unknown proportion of topsoil. It's in the wrong place and is doing damage both to the environment that it came from and the environment it is going to, and it's not natural for this to occur.

Humans have played a major part in setting the whole cycle in motion. If people had not cut down the forest cover and overstocked the pasture in Eastland, Cyclone Bola could have come and gone having knocked down lots of trees, but leaving most of the soil in place; new seedlings would have started growing within weeks.

At the height of another flood in February 2004, Dr Troy Baisden and his colleagues at Landcare Research took samples from the swollen Manawatu River as it passed under the Fitzherbert Bridge in Palmerston North. They reported that at the peak of the flood, 28 tonnes of sediment per second was going past the bridge, a quarter of which was rich topsoil. That is equivalent to a fleet of 170 ten-tonne truckloads a minute driving by. If you've ever done any landscaping you'll appreciate the implications of this — truckloads of topsoil do not come cheap.

In cases like these, some of the soil remains suspended in the river, doing damage to the freshwater ecosystem for months, if not years. The rest gets washed out to the coastal area where it silts up the most productive part of the sea. Yes, chopping down trees does result in fewer fish to catch. This is another of those flow-on effects ('down-streaming' both literally and in business-speak) where the connection is not immediately obvious to us, so we make the assumption that it is not there. This has all the common sense of a small child covering his eyes and saying: 'You can't see me.'

All of these little things that we can't see add up and are playing a major part in the destruction of our environment, yet they are rarely mentioned in national waste management plans.

Of course, New Zealand is not alone in the loss of topsoil. Our nearest neighbor, Australia, loses millions of tonnes of soil each year as it is blown off drought-ravaged land into the sea, with some of it crossing the Tasman Sea to New Zealand. When sufficient topsoil has gone, the next stage is the formation of dust storms from the remaining layers. In one dust storm on 24 and 25 May 1994 in South Australia, a scientific team reported in the *Australian Journal of Soil and Water Conservation* that the weight of dust in the plume had been eight million tonnes.

American topsoil loss is reported to be in the range of three to seven billion tons annually — this in a country well aware of the hardships created by dustbowl conditions in the 1930s, when people in great swathes of the Midwest were forced off their farms and moved to California.

In the 1960s, in the height of the Soviet era, Kazakhstan produced as much grain as Canada and Australia combined. However, this was not to last, because the soil was never suited to such intensive cultivation techniques. Now this area is a dustbowl and may make the transition from semi-arid land to arid and become a desert. The same phenomenon is now occurring in China, where dust storms from the encroaching desert regularly close Beijing airport and force city-dwellers to wear face masks. Ditto in North Africa.

As Jared Diamond points out in his seminal history of human civilisation *Guns, Germs and Steel*, modern society first evolved in a lush, forested area known to historians as the 'Fertile Triangle', which has subsequently turned into the deserts of the Middle East.

Personally, as businesspeople we have high regard for the importance of free enterprise and competition. But we are certain that market forces alone will not resolve these big issues until it is too late. The current market overvalues speed and efficiency and has little appreciation or understanding of solutions that are a bit slower — like, for example, methodically planting lots of trees in the right places (more on this later). With all of the above challenges there are some surprisingly simple solutions, but they involve vision, leadership and commitment from national and local governments. The great thing about democracy is that we get to decide who's sitting in those chairs, making those vital decisions.

Toxic waste

Having documented two substantial sources of waste that have slipped through the net for planning purposes, it's worth looking for any other significant waste streams which might need examination. Several can be identified.

Mining waste is a massive but uncertain volume of material in almost every country on earth. In many cases it has far more hazardous components than exist in household waste, yet it rarely features in waste analyses. On 30 January 2000, the tailings dam at a mine in Baia Mare, Romania, half owned by the Australian mining company Esmeralda Exploration Ltd, spilled 378,000 tons of cyanide-contaminated waste into the Danube River. It caused one of the worst river pollution incidents Europe has ever seen, killing all aquatic life for kilometres. Defective disposal of mine tailings (fine-grained processing residues) blight many countries and can be expected to cause problems for decades — quite possibly centuries. In *Collapse*, Jared Diamond describes the nightmarish multi-billion-dollar difficulties involved in cleaning up abandoned mine sites in the US.

Australia has an ongoing problem with drought, yet it discharges 1325 billion litres of sewage and waste water into the ocean every year. Annual discharges into the oceans of rubbish from ships and lost fishing gear amount worldwide to 200 million tonnes, a figure similar to the amount of waste sent to landfill in the United States. If the figure seems a bit high, you might care to consider that to start with, 10,000 shipping containers and their contents are lost overboard every year. Anything that floats ends up caught in a vortex of ocean currents called gyres and moves towards the centre, where it remains trapped and slowly decomposes as the plastic components photo-degrade into smaller particles. The North Pacific gyre is about the size of the continental United States and is littered with plastic junk to a depth of 30 m. At the centre, the gyre contains six times as many particles of plastic as zooplankton, the bottom of the oceanic food chain. To make matters worse, the decomposing plastic molecules are blotters for other pollutants such as PCBs and pesticides, so that far from being inert they become the zing in our seafood cocktail.

Allied to the problem of waste discharged into the marine environment is the discharge of ships' ballast water, taken on board in one place and emptied elsewhere complete with its load of alien animal life, which displaces less vigorous local species to the detriment of the local ecosystem.

And so it goes with waste problems, ad infinitum it sometimes seems. According to an *Economist* report in July 2003, contaminated water is blamed for something close to 60 per cent of all human illness, killing 12,000 people daily — an annual total of 4.38 million, greater than the entire New Zealand population. It makes for grim reading, doesn't it? But don't lose hope. There are solutions.

The solutions

We've outlined enough to show that waste is a big issue, and while putting out the recycling bin or composting our kitchen scraps makes an important contribution, it's not ever going to touch some of the really big things that are building up to bite us. Captain Charles Moore, who studied the waste in the North Pacific gyre and reported his findings to the Global Marine Litter Information Gateway, says he would not be surprised to see a ten-fold increase in the quantity of waste in this location in the next ten years. We asked Richard Tong, an Auckland environmental scientist who has specialised in recycling and who provided much of the research for Part Three of this book, for his recommended solutions to these problems. His answer is as follows:

> In 1976 I had just finished a master's degree in zoology at the University of Auckland and was fed up with looking down a microscope, so I approached my local council with ideas for a recycling scheme. This initiative coincided with a push by a group of environmental organisations to improve waste management in the broader Auckland region. Jeanette Fitzsimmons, now

an MP and co-leader of the New Zealand Green Party, was a key figure in one of these organisations and everything came together with the birth of the Devonport Recycling Scheme in 1977 — the first in New Zealand and the model for many developments overseas. I was the first Recycling Officer employed in this country and have spent 30 years honing my skills, consulting in the environmental field in New Zealand and around the world.

I know that the issues are huge and while we are making little headway at the moment, the openings are there to deal with them because there's enormous enthusiasm and goodwill towards the environment. I remember a lovely story that Jeanette used to cite. She had returned to New Zealand in the mid 1970s with a couple of young children after some time in Switzerland, where she had seen recycling in action. Whenever she mentioned that recycling worked in Switzerland, people would say: 'Ah, but the Swiss are different.' After the Devonport scheme met with nearly universal approval and economic success and Jeanette told people that it was working in Devonport, they would say: 'Ah, but people in Devonport are different.' I have now seen operations all over North America and Europe, and implemented initiatives as far apart as rural New Zealand and Vietnam, and can assure you that people share the same enthusiasm for recycling wherever you go.

The first step is that we need to decide, and then articulate, what we think is good and what is bad in the environmental context. Most societies have decided that smoking is bad and have started on the path towards eliminating it. If we agree that irresponsible waste disposal is bad — and this seems to be the consensus — then we should say so and act accordingly. We should not have councils that negotiate bulk deals because they want to make dumping waste cheap, or others that pay contractors extra for handling more waste — thus giving them an incentive to increase the amount of waste going to landfill.

We should impose a levy on every tonne of waste that goes for disposal and that should increase according to a simple formula every year. Then everyone knows that the bad behavior costs more than the good behaviour and that the gap will widen. No smoker is under the illusion that cigarettes will be cheaper next year.

Then there is the penalty end of the spectrum. I believe that we need to impose long prison terms on serious environmental offenders. Taiwan has looked at life imprisonment for contaminating groundwater and I think that's of the right order — again, a clear, straightforward message.

The next important step is to sort out hazardous wastes of all categories and in all countries. A New Zealand Department of Health report in 1982 emphasised the need for more adequate record-keeping and improved management of hazardous wastes; this has still not been fully implemented.

I would like to see cities in the affluent world become twins with less affluent ones, and for the wealthy twin to cover the cost of specific clean-up and environmental education campaigns overseas. These would be funded from waste levies so that the bad action in the rich country, dumping, covers the good activity, clean-up, in the poorer one.

Finally, there is an answer that will ensure a start is made with one of the biggest issues, need not cost a fortune and can be applied anywhere. We know that topsoil loss and desertification are huge problems involving massive numbers. At the same time, organic waste makes up about half of traditional waste in most parts of the world. By the simple action of composting this and supplying it to nurseries we can create a virtuous cycle where trees are raised, planted and nurtured to minimise erosion and topsoil loss and absorb greenhouse gases at the same time. This integrated operation should also be funded by waste levies to drive home the good and bad environmental messages with appropriate economic ones.

There are two examples from history that we think are relevant here, with the first attributed to Napoleon. Allegedly, he had issued an order to plant more trees to provide wood to construct an enhanced navy. When one of his minions pointed out that this initiative would take hundreds of years to be successful, Napoleon is said to have replied: 'Well, that is the very reason to start this afternoon.' A century later, Gandhi made the observation that the government of India could never plant enough trees to prevent deforestation, but if it could persuade every Indian to plant one tree then forests would emerge.

We are all capable of digging one or two holes and planting a couple of trees. We have to choose the right species, plant them in the right places, and ensure that sure they are nurtured and their future secured, but these are all things we can manage. The challenge for our decision-makers is to ensure this is a top priority.

With regard to the earlier statistics on wastewater contamination, it's worth mentioning that in November 1980 the United Nations launched a Decade on Water. Meeting the goals set then on the supply of clean fresh water and sanitation would mean that from now until 2015, 400,000 people every day would have to be provided with adequate sanitation. This figure gives new meaning to stories about the difficulty of finding a plumber but it is not as daunting as it may seem. WHO statistics show that during the 1980s a remarkable 438,000 connections to clean, fresh water were established *daily* worldwide — an effort which saved the lives of well over a hundred million people.

Chapter 13 contains actions you can take starting today to minimise the waste you, your family and your business create.

Having started this chapter in outer space we may as well leave the discussion of waste on the same theme. There are about a million bits of space junk orbiting the Earth. According to the BBC, all but 9000 of these are smaller than a postage stamp but are still capable of doing damage to a spacecraft because of the speed at which they are travelling. When zipping by at 36,000 km per hour, a metal sphere the size of a tennis ball packs the same punch as 25 sticks of explosive. It would be a most unfortunate irony if, in the future, having finally realised that we had made an irreparable mess of the environment on this planet, we set off to colonise space only to be hit by a piece of space junk on the way.

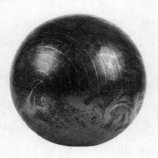

11 | people and money

We write this while working in Sao Paulo, Brazil, a city of almost 20 million people, a population as big as Australia's. It's rained the past few days, so from our roof we can view a surreal landscape of buildings, stretching as far as the eye can see in any direction. Flying in, you get a sense that this city goes on forever, with no discernable centre — endless, seething humanity.

It's to feed the growth of this metropolis that the subject of our childhood myth and *awe*, the great Amazon jungle, is being steadily transformed into a bland wasteland of industrial cattle and soy farming.

You can't blame the Brazilians; people in the developing world only want what the rest of us have, for decades, taken for granted, and we have to find ways to sustain that. What humanity can't afford is to keep creating more and more Sao Paulos.

In the UK, the 2007 report of the All-Party Parliamentary Group on Population, Development and Reproductive Health stated that unless contraception was put back at the top of the agenda for international efforts to alleviate global poverty, the UN Millennium Development Goals would be missed, leading to an 'unsustainable' 10.5 billion world population by 2050.

The belief promoted by some politicians and businessmen that more people will create stronger economies through increased demand and cheap labour availability is ill conceived and will ultimately lead to collapse. For example, in *The Future Eaters* Tim Flannery rejects ideas of a 50–100 million population for Australia by arguing that the country's long-term 'natural carrying capacity' may, in fact, be more like 6–12 million — lower than even its current 20 million. He suggests that Australia is setting up its future generations for disaster by spending the proceeds of finite resources on subsidising current deficits.

The British report describes the 90s as a 'lost decade' in which other priorities moved up the agenda. It also states that world leaders must reject neo-conservative religious ideologies that have recently forced non-governmental organisations outside America to choose between promoting family planning and receiving US funds. Religious policies around childbirth originated in past eras of extremely high child mortality, when the survival of a tribe depended on maintaining a high birth rate. Unfortunately, these have the opposite consequence under modern conditions. Furthermore, any 21st century 'tribe' aiming to gain dominance by out-populating its rivals creates a likelihood that at the end of the struggle there will be nothing left worth owning.

In the long run, population is perhaps the biggest of all sustainability issues. As explained in the introduction to this book, we are already consuming 25 per cent more resources than this planet can produce, and by 2050 that figure is forecast to be 200 per cent.

Affluenza

In October 2006 the population of the United States passed the 300 million mark, having reached the 200 million milestone just 39 years earlier, in 1967. The American Census Bureau estimates that one baby is born in the USA every eight seconds, one person dies every 12 seconds and a new immigrant settles in the country every 31 seconds. This amounts to a net increase, on average, of one person every 14 seconds.

In other words, there are an extra 6171 Americans every day or 2.25 million every year. However, the extra people do not bring their own geography. Their needs and the strain their demands place on the environment join those of the existing population.

America has inspired the world with its material achievements, but at the cost of using vastly more energy and resources than any other group of people on the planet.

We've calculated that in 2003 we and our friends in New Zealand used energy equivalent to 347.1 kg of oil (kgoe) to fuel our residential lives; our American friends used 923.5 kgoe in the same year. Nothing we have seen suggests that consuming this extra energy provides them with any additional fun or happiness. There is, in fact, some evidence to the contrary. In general, Americans are more sedentary, more obese and less active than their forebears, who did a lot more for themselves and were probably happier for it.

The story of energy use reappears in just about every measure of human impact on the environment. American demand for fresh water from rivers, dams and lakes is reaching a breaking point — the available water in the Colorado River, for instance, has been allocated many times over.

Nowhere is this disproportionate global footprint summarised better than in housing. The average US house has doubled in size since 1950 while at the same time the size of the average family has been dropping. In 1950 each individual had 27 square metres of house to themselves, but by 2003 this had increased to 83 square metres per person. This three-fold increase in house size per person is a remarkable vindication of the observation by the American essayist Ralph Waldo Emerson (1803–1882) that 'much will have more'.

Lest anyone think we're taking a swipe at the US, let's all be quite clear that the rest of the world is trying desperately to follow in America's footsteps. Houses in New Zealand have doubled in size in the same period — not to the extent witnessed in the States, but that's only a measure of the relative affluence of our two countries and not the dreams or aspirations of New Zealanders.

Another prescient observation was made by the brilliant American economist and statesman John Kenneth Galbraith (1908–2006), who concluded his 1961 book *The Affluent Society* with the words: 'To furnish a barren room is one thing. To continue to crowd in furniture until the foundation buckles is quite another. To have failed to solve the problem of producing goods would have been to continue man in his oldest and most grievous misfortune. But to fail to see that we have solved it, and to fail to proceed thence to the next task, would be fully as tragic.'

Galbraith was one of the first to identify modern over-consumption, even before it emerged as today's extreme excesses. Universally, people are aspiring to the trappings of modern consumer lifestyles and more and more of them are realising the dream. On May 12th 2000 a girl named Assar (meaning hope) was born in a slum in New Delhi, India, and was named as the one billionth Indian, as part of a government family-planning promotion. With India joining China in the billion-plus population club, we start to see the effect of some really big numbers.

The China Modernisation Report 2006 prepared by the Chinese Academy of Sciences predicted continued dramatic increases in Chinese economic activity and a surge in the ownership of consumer items such as motor vehicles. It said half of China's people would own cars by 2050. What will the world be like with double or treble the present number of cars on the road?

The Canadian military analyst and internationally syndicated columnist Gwynne Dyer observed that: 'Somewhere between now and the future it [China] envisages for 2050, the negative consequences of continuing down the present path will become so large and undeniable that the present development pattern will be abandoned.'

But Dyer also noted that: 'On the other hand, the day must arrive when the people of China, India, Brazil and Indonesia live as well as Americans, or else there will be hell to pay. So the day may well arrive when more than half of all Americans don't own cars either. The future, as usual, is not going to be like the present.'

In the decades ahead, these soaring economies will place ever-greater demands on existing resources, with profound implications for the environment locally, regionally and globally.

The links between the environment — as both a source of raw materials and as a sink for the wastes from human activity — and the economy present a complex set of interactions in their own right. This complexity can be illustrated by a simple example with very far-reaching implications. In 2005, China manufactured 40 million internal combustion engines. Six million of these went into locally made trucks and automobiles, part of China's emerging challenge to the world's auto industry. When used, these vehicles will clearly produce greenhouse gases and contribute to climate change, but the other 34 million engines may pose a greater and far more immediate environmental challenge.

The majority of them are small in size and are running generators and pumps in China, India and in other less industrialised nations around the world. Using fossil fuel for energy, the pumps are extracting fossil groundwater for agricultural irrigation and small-scale use. The use of this form of groundwater, which was put in place during the last Ice Age and is not replenished like water in normal aquifers, has been a major, if little-noticed, environmental concern for decades. *New Scientist* reports that in the past, the extraction was limited to officially sanctioned bores, but the explosion of small pumps has given every farmer with a modest amount of capital access to the necessary technology.

There is concern that this may be threatening the achievements of the green revolution when agricultural yields throughout Asia, in particular, were dramatically increased by a combination of new varieties of grain, fertiliser and irrigation. According to *New Scientist*, there is the added concern that much of the increased pumping in river deltas in Asia is causing them to sink, with the prospect that the homes, farms, villages and towns of over six million people will sink under the sea by 2050.

To be sure, technological advances will mitigate some of these risks. In January 2007, for instance, the Co-operative Research Centre for the Plant-Based Management of Dryland Salinity in West Australia announced that researchers from the universities of West Australia and Adelaide have developed a new wheat strain that can be sown on moderately salt-affected soils, containing up to one quarter the salt levels of sea water. This breakthrough has been reached using conventional plant-breeding techniques and not genetic engineering, and will allow Australian farmers to raise grain on an extra 600,000 hectares of the grain belt that have been affected by agricultural salinisation.

However, as Flannery argues in *The Future Eaters*: 'There is no doubt that technology has had some impact, but thus far it has been insufficient to reverse environmental degradation. Although it may well happen, it is of little value to assume that technology will solve these problems. This is because if we make assumptions about future change in such areas, we create a hypothetical species; one that might exist if only we could change our habits.'

Changing our habits is something we must do, despite the difficulties. Gross over-consumption is a very important part of the globesity problem and it will only be seriously tackled when we collectively realise the true scale and urgency of the problem. On a personal level, we all face the challenge of undoing years of conditioning that told us more is better and bigger is best. In Chapter 13 we list some practical steps you can take to make a difference in this arena.

The challenge of sheer overpopulation is even thornier but we have to face it now also, to improve our chances of successfully facing the others. Borders won't insulate us from ecological disasters *or* economic ones in today's globalised world. Nor will Star Wars defence systems protect us from a multi-million-strong horde of desperate global refugees. Flannery, this time in *The Weathermakers*, quotes a Pentagon-commissioned report as follows: 'Humans fight when they outstrip the carrying capacity of their environment . . . Every time there is a choice between starving and raiding, humans raid.'

At the same time as encouraging technological and conservationist solutions to our current problems, we need to place population at the top of world political and religious agendas. Without this, we will simply increase the scale of our other sustainability challenges and — at best — bequeath yet another nightmare to our grandchildren.

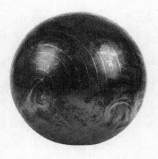

12 | water, water everywhere?

We have clear memories of the pictures of our serene blue planet beamed back by the astronauts on Apollo 8 in 1968. This was the first time we had seen ourselves from the outside, and the images were both beautiful and moving.

At first glance they showed only one thing: water. Around 71 per cent of our planet's surface area is covered with water, and 97 per cent of that is salt water. Of the three per cent that is not salty, 90 per cent of it is locked up — at least for now — in the Antarctic ice sheet or as buried groundwater. The stuff that comes out of our taps at home, irrigates our agriculture and provides the water for industry comprises only a miniscule 0.3 per cent of all the water on the planet.

Life on Earth exists because of two physical components: topsoil and water. Topsoil is the combination of all the physical nutrients contributed by weathered rocks from aeons past, combined with the decayed remains of previous fungal, plant and animal inhabitants. Without water this mix would be useless, but with it magic starts to happen. The Hungarian Nobel Laureate Dr Albert Szent-Gyorgy called water the 'matrix of life' for its remarkable properties as a solvent, dissolving more compounds than any other. It also makes up a staggering two thirds of each of our bodies.

Physiologists liken our bodies to containers filled with bags of seawater. We need fresh water to regulate the salinity inside each bag and more to move nutrients and energy to the cells in each bag. Yet more fresh water is then needed to remove the waste produced by burning that energy. Quite simply, if there is no water, there is no life. It's for this reason that the first thing NASA does on missions to other worlds is to look for evidence of water.

There are only a limited number of sources of the water we need. It can either come from rainfall collected directly off our roof or, more likely, as surface water collected in a natural or man-made water storage like a dam. Alternatively, it can come from a river, which might have its source in melting snow on mountains miles away, or it can be pumped up from an aquifer, which is basically an underground river or lake. Each of these systems is part of a giant water cycle, in which some of the water used for irrigation evaporates into the atmosphere to come down as rain somewhere else. It slowly works its way into groundwater to recharge an aquifer and, in some cases, takes an immense underground journey before resurfacing as a natural spring. We have already mentioned that the springs that resupply Lake Taupo, in the centre of the North Island, take a phenomenal 80 years to recharge.

There is one more important source of water for humanity and that is fossil groundwater: water that was captured in vast subterranean cavities during earlier ice ages, which is not replenished by normal cycles. Fossil groundwater, pumped to the surface by machines running on fossil fuels, has played a crucial part in the agricultural productivity of all of the major grain-growing areas of the world, and these water reserves are being depleted at an alarming rate.

We'll look at an example of a depleted fossil groundwater reserve later, but first let's acknowledge that most of you reading this book will not have suffered from a lack of water in your lifetime, other than perhaps a sprinkler ban during the summer months. The idea that we might run out of water seems like a problem from a futuristic sci-fi film (think *Mad Max*) but for many living on our planet the quest for enough water to sustain daily life is a constant struggle.

There are simple actions we can all take to help, some of which are laid out in Chapter 13 (for a comprehensive list, read the remarkable 'Aqueous Solutions' chapter in *Natural Capitalism* by Paul Hawken, Amory Lovins and L. Hunter Lovins). But for now, let's take a look at some of the general problems related to water supply.

Nor any drop to drink

Over 1.1 billion people, one in six folk on the planet today, have no access to adequate supplies of clean water. This usually results in women or children having to walk kilometres each day to collect a modest amount, then carry it home. Water experts have decided that we each need an absolute minimum of 20 to 50 litres a day — one or two bucketfuls.

At the other end of the spectrum 2.6 billion people, or one in 2.5 people, have no access to sanitation. It is self-evident that the absence of adequate sanitation will inevitably threaten the remaining supplies of clean fresh water. As mentioned in Chapter 10, contaminated water is blamed for something close to 60 per cent of all human illness, killing 12,000 people daily or an annual total of 4.38 million: greater than the entire New Zealand population.

A quick look at the situation in China will bring these mind-boggling numbers down to earth with a crunch. The first problem facing China is a national scarcity of water resources, having only a quarter of the global average to start with. Starting from that point is bad enough, but the scarcity is much worse in some parts of the country than others. In northern China, the supply of water is as low as 10 per cent of the global average. The north is home to 47 per cent of China's population, produces 45 per cent of its GDP and accounts for 65 per cent of China's cultivated land. It has only 19 per cent of the country's water resources, and in 2004 it was reported that the water supply level across northern China was at three quarters of the recommended 20-50 litres a day minimum level. On the North China Plain, they were down to half the recommended minimum.

As if this situation was not bad enough, 75 per cent of the water in question comes from wells that are abstracting fossil groundwater, which is not being replenished. The water is not being treated, does not meet minimum WHO standards for drinking water and, to top the situation off, the wastewater of only 310 larger Chinese cities is treated in any way. The wastes from the other 669 larger cities and 17,000 smaller towns is being discharged untreated into nearby watercourses. The burden of waterborne illness and disease in parts of China is massive.

The city of Harbin in north China used to be famous for its ice sculptures in winter, but it hit the headlines in November 2005 when a huge chemical spill left its four million inhabitants without drinking water. For weeks the world watched the progress of the chemical slick as it passed across China and into Russia. This turned out to be one of those 'tip of the iceberg' events. Pan Yue, deputy head of the State Environmental Protection Administration (SEPA), is reported in *Time* magazine to have confirmed that 130 other spills took place throughout the country that year, or *one every three days*.

In 1972 the Yellow River ran dry for the first time because of the volume of water being taken upstream. In 1999 it was dry for seven months. Eighty percent of China's seven major river systems no longer support fish. It is easy to see why Pan Yue regularly warns of the possibility of an environmental catastrophe — confronted with these alarming facts, it would appear to be a question of when rather than if one or more major traumas will occur.

In this dire situation, all is not lost. China has the financial reserves to make a significant dent in these problems, and has simply not yet marshalled the concerted political will to make a significant start. Commentators suggest that officials at a local level are too keen to line their own pockets or maintain the economic boom to take seriously the leads from central government to reduce the extent of pollution. One way or another, this must surely soon change.

But if the Chinese have a water supply plight, then consider the situation in India, which has about 20 per cent less water than China. In Kenya they have to get by on less than half of the minimum required water per person, and areas like the Seychelles and the West Bank somehow manage with no internal water resources whatsoever. With an average US daily usage of around 5000 litres per person (including a domestic usage of 450 litres), ranking sixth highest in the world behind New Zealand in first place, hopefully we in the West won't have to reach a similar state before changing our wasteful ways.

In one end . . .

The problem of water availability and adequate sanitation is not limited to the adequacy or otherwise of the resource, or even to the quality of the water, although that is obviously critical. Amory Lovins, the energy guru we mentioned earlier and founder of the Rocky Mountain Institute, states that two thirds of the electricity consumed worldwide is used to power motors, the majority of which are used for pumping fluids such as water. Providing a sustainable energy infrastructure to deliver clean water and remove wastewater is as much a part of the water issue as the resource itself.

There are 500 major rivers in the world, and half of them are severely depleted or polluted. As we have seen in China, very often they suffer both indignities. A century ago, before we developed wastewater treatment technologies in the West, even with some intensively polluting industrial and mining activities, the figure was only 10 per cent of this number.

But there's always hope. The Great Lakes between Canada and the United States were in a very grim state for most of the twentieth century, with so much oil in and on the water that on more than one occasion entire bays or rivers caught fire. The Great Lakes Basin ecosystem is the largest freshwater system in the world and contains 20 per cent of the world's available freshwater. Thanks to the Herculean efforts of cooperative agencies at the national, state, provincial and local levels the situation is now improving for most of the environmental indicators measured.

New technological threats

Similar success stories can be recorded for the Thames in England and the Seine, Danube and Rhine in Europe. Each has required gargantuan efforts over decades but significant progress has ultimately been made. In all of these cases, however, the story gets more complicated the deeper we look.

Water clean-up efforts involve diverting major sources of waste to prevent them from contaminating waterways, including untreated human waste from urban centres, industrial wastes and agricultural run-off. Having mastered these we find that there are new classes of waste that we had not dreamt of a decade or two earlier.

Samples of drinking water taken in Europe or North America often contain trace quantities of commonly used pharmaceuticals, for example the antidepressant Prozac. These compounds are appearing because they've been designed to pack a punch in the recipient's body and resist its attempts to break them down, so they wind up in water treatment works and can ultimately circulate back out to other water users. They are generally present in trace quantities not expected to have any impact on adults, but might raise a concern for developing children in the future.

A potentially greater catastrophe may come from the recently developed science of nano-particles, which are being used in such diverse products as cosmetics, sunscreens, tennis rackets and car paint. These particles are so tiny that they can easily pass through the skin, lung and in some cases blood-brain barriers. They have been found to cause brain damage and genetic changes in fish, and have been named as a future environmental disaster possibly worse than asbestos. (There are still 3000 deaths per year from decades-old asbestos, long after it was banned.) Commercial goals seem to be taking precedence over methodical scientific prudence around this technology at present. As with genetically modified organisms, regulation is desperately needed in this field.

Some of these new problems might be beaten by new clean-up technologies. New Zealander Professor Terry Collins is the director of the Institute for Green Oxidation Chemistry at Carnegie Mellon University in the United States. In 1999 he received the Presidential Green Chemistry Challenge Award for 20 years' research leading to the development of TAML hydrogen peroxide activators. These are being used to revolutionise the bleaching processes in the pulp and paper industries and show promise in cleaning up other contaminants like the pharmaceuticals now being found in natural waters. However, it is early days and these developments provide no reason to retreat from desperately needed environmental protection efforts.

The best of intentions

If it is not enough that a lack of available water resources and contamination with waste water and industrial pollutants plague so many Third World countries, in some instances we, in the First World, have offered help yet made things worse. In an effort to reduce high levels of infant mortality from waterborne disease in Bangladesh, UNICEF and the World Bank supported projects to drill millions of deep tube wells in the Ganges Delta area to provide clean water. This project, which ran through the 1970s and 80s, chopped infant mortality and the incidence of diarrhoeal diseases in half but, unexpectedly, left a legacy of arsenic poisoning for tens of millions of people. The tube wells had tapped into a body of deeper groundwater where there were high levels of naturally occurring arsenic. Further overseas aid efforts to remove the arsenic using filters have been widely reported to have failed, as the equipment was too complex for the rural setting, but the overall problem is now being tackled by a combination of simple, locally designed filters and boring into even deeper groundwater where the arsenic deposits have been leached out by other geological processes.

The lessons to the foreign aid community have been clearly learnt: to avoid grand-scale, single-fix solutions; to continually monitor progress (some initial testing for arsenic suggested it was at acceptable levels but the testing did not continue), and to involve locals in the design of solutions that suit their particular setting.

New hope around agricultural abuse

The best news in the water pollution stakes is in the water use game. The greediest water user, worldwide, is agricultural irrigation, taking around 70 per cent of all freshwater taken for human use. With very few exceptions, the methods of irrigation in use are wasteful of both water and soil nutrients, using one precious resource to flush the other away. In other cases we are over-supplying water to crops only to have it evaporate.

In some areas there are still subsidies to irrigate, providing financial assistance with pumping infrastructure and energy costs or agricultural subsidies on crops produced. Clearly these subsidies need to be aligned with the best practice from the perspective of water-resource use as well as agricultural method. The whole lot then needs to be examined in the context of climate change.

Again, there are no universal quick-fix solutions, but through education in the latest agricultural techniques, tailor-made for each area, we can lower the demand for water dramatically and also reduce pollution from agricultural activities. Certainly the effort is going in at the policy-making end, with international workshops now occurring on a regular basis.

The Aquastat service developed by the Water and Agriculture Division of the Food and Agricultural Organisation (FAO) of the United Nations has information on every water-related variable you could imagine, for countries many of us have not heard of. This service is a clear example of the practical benefits of universal access to the internet. We might suffer from information overload, but getting practical stuff to a farmer relating to his region and his river is wonderful stuff. Take a look at *www.fao.org/ag/agl/aglw/aquastat/ dbases/index.stm* and gain heart for the future about what we can do when we put our minds to it.

The United Nations declared 2003 to be the International Year of Fresh Water. In March 2003, the World Water Forum in Kyoto, Japan and again, in June 2003, the G8 Summit in Evian, France, both reaffirmed the UN's goals. But before we celebrate too loudly we should remember that on November 10 1980 the General Assembly of the United Nations devoted a day to launch the United Nations Decade on Water, and 27 years later more people than ever are in a desperate situation. However, as noted in Chapter 10, in the 1980s we did achieve a remarkable 438,000 connections to clean freshwater daily, worldwide, and the record suggests that that effort saved the lives of well over a hundred million people. Hopefully this time we will finish the job.

The price to pay

The issue of subsidies has already been raised and this highlights the underlying issues related to water which are receiving attention all over the world: its value, and whether access to it is a universal human right or a commodity to be traded. Having woken up to the idea that water is a valuable resource and, certainly in some places, very scarce, businesspeople and politicians have realised that often no one is getting charged for it, or if they are they are getting it far too cheap. In some settings, because there's been no charge there's been limited provision for upgrading the infrastructure, and vast amounts of water are being lost through leaks. At the consumer end the suggestion has been made that because they do not have to pay, consumers place no value on water and are wasteful in its use — and that maybe privatising the resource offers the rigor of scrutiny by the marketplace.

We believe that all players have valid contributions to make, and that we need to develop a regime that suits each local setting, ensuring that everyone realises that water must not be wasted and at the same time guaranteeing that no one is ever deprived of their minimum entitlement. One possible solution might be a graduated charging system that gives everyone a basic entitlement and provides for larger volumes to be available to heavy users, at a price.

● | BOTTLED WATER

As people involved in the fitness industry, we can't leave this subject without mentioning the massive commerce that's grown up around bottled water. Some have singled it out as a huge consumer con, but we're not quite so unkind.

We mentioned in Chapter 5 some of the benefits and some possible health risks associated with plastic containers and the lack of purity standards for bottled water. But from a personal health perspective, it's a lot better to drink water than anything else, so if we're going to drink something from a bottle then it's best to be water.

From the planetary perspective, however, we must regretfully say that we need a lot fewer bottles in the environment. And you know from your own experience how often you buy bottled water and how infrequently you use those same bottles again. We'd like to diminish the energy demands of producing and delivering billions of small bottles of water all over the world in planes, trucks and cars, only 20 per cent of which are then estimated to be recycled.

If you'd like to help with this effort, or you're concerned about the quality of water in your area, then consider investing in a water filter for your home or workplace or carrying a reusable bottle.

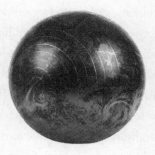

13 | it comes from in here

So what can you do? What possible difference can you as an individual, one of six and a half billion people living on Earth, really make? As we explained in our Introduction, solving the sustainability crisis involves unprecedented acts of government — beginning with the most urgent problem of global warming. Vital legislation must be pushed through, despite powerful corporate lobbying, and everyone is required to act in order to protect our planet.

It's a time for selflessness, positive action and generosity — especially by those of us who can most afford it. We are the ones in the strongest position to fix this problem. Those who can't, won't, and therefore those of us who can, must.

We're not much enamoured with ecological footprint calculators — they tend to emphasise the negative rather than show the huge positive differences we can make by adjusting our lives. But they do give a good overall picture of who is responsible for the mess we're in. For example, when Jackie and I enter our details into one of the most respected international calculators, Global

Footprint Network *(www.footprintnetwork.org)*, we're told that we're each responsible for approximately 14 hectares of land use (a hectare is around the size of two football fields), against a global availability of 1.8 hectares per person. We're also told that if everyone lived like us, we'd need approximately eight planets to sustain the present world population. Even cutting out the huge amount of air travel we do in our jobs would only get us down to the national average for our country of 8.7 hectares and five planets. Ouch.

The important thing here is not to feel guilty about the situation, but to get on with doing something about it. As Amory Lovins said in a 2005 article in *Scientific American:* 'The climate problem was created by millions of bad decisions over decades, but climate stability can be restored by millions of sensible choices — buying a more efficient lamp or car, adding insulation or caulk to your home, repealing subsidies for waste and rewarding desired outcomes.'

There's a wonderful moment in *An Inconvenient Truth* when Al Gore shows the current increases in the levels of carbon and where we're headed in the next 50 years. It's a horrifying sight as carbon emissions continue to rise unabated. Then, he shows what would happen if we changed certain things. Bit by bit, the carbon emissions *actually fall.* It's the moment in the film where you take a deep breath and think: 'We can beat this.' As Gore says, we have the technology available, right now, to save the planet.

To quote Tim Flannery: 'You can, in a few months rather than the 50 years allowed by some governments, easily attain the 70 per cent reduction in emissions required to stabilise the Earth's climate. All it takes are a few changes to your personal life, none of which requires serious sacrifices.'

The following is our list of the actions we can take to accomplish this. Every list you read has a different order of priorities; we believe the aim should be to do the things you are capable of, at the greatest speed you can afford. There's a nice kind of serendipity at work here, as most of these actions have the double benefit of not only contributing to planetary health but also improving your personal life or that of your family or business.

Increase your understanding

Knowledge builds motivation and empowerment, and you'll achieve better results if you focus your energies in the right direction. Read the great authors on sustainability and the topics surrounding it. Certain books have dramatically changed our lives and those of friends we have shared them with. We have mentioned some of them in earlier chapters. We believe the most essential are:

- *The Weathermakers* by Tim Flannery — in our view the gold standard on global warming. An internationally acclaimed scientist and 2007 Australian of the Year, Professor Flannery's books are fascinating to read. He has also written other environmental masterpieces such as *The Future Eaters: An Ecological History of the Australasian Lands and People* and *The Eternal Frontier: An Ecological History of North America and Its Peoples.*

- Our close favourite on global warming is *Heat: How to Stop the Planet Burning* by leading UK journalist George Monbiot. He provides convincing arguments for even stronger and more urgent solutions than other commentators.

- *Collapse: How Societies Choose to Fail or Survive* by Jared Diamond is a consummate overview of our present sustainability challenges, based on detailed comparisons with human civilisations throughout history that have collapsed or survived for ecological reasons. Another of the world's greatest scientists, Diamond writes books which, like Flannery's, are fascinating to read and will enormously expand your world view (his other works include *Guns, Germs and Steel: The Fates of Human Societies* and *The Third Chimpanzee: The Evolution and Future of the Human Animal).*

- *The Omnivore's Dilemma* by Michael Pollan clearly and beautifully explains the effects of industrial agriculture on our bodies and the ecosystem. This book will empower you to significantly improve both the environment and your health through small adjustments in your shopping habits. Pollan is a clever and original writer whose other ecologically oriented works include *The Botany of Desire: A Plant's-Eye View of the World.* Our other favorites in this area include Jane Goodall's *Harvest for Hope* and *The Ethics of What We Eat* by Peter Singer and Jim Mason, plus, of course, some of the great cookbooks we mentioned in Chapter 5.

- *Natural Capitalism: The Next Industrial Revolution* by Paul Hawken, Amory B Lovins and LH Lovins is the ultimate book on green business. This brilliant compilation contains a variety of solutions to every sustainability problem. As Bill Clinton says on the cover, it 'proves beyond any argument that there are presently available technologies, and those just on the horizon, which will permit us to get richer by cleaning, not by spoiling, the environment'. It's a must-read for everyone in business and government, with lots of great practical ideas for individuals as well.

- Environmental classics, some of which are still on our future reading list, include Mark Reisner's *Cadillac Desert: The American West and its Disappearing Water, Small is Beautiful: A Study of Economics as if People Mattered* by EF Schumacher, *The Closing Circle: Nature, Man, and Technology* by Barry Commoner, the works of David Suzuki and of Paul and Anne Ehrlich; *Gaia: A New Look at Life on Earth* by James Lovelock, and the 1960s book credited with kick-starting the modern environmental movement, *Silent Spring* by Rachel Carson.

- From the politicians' corner we enjoyed Mikhail Gorbachev's *Manifesto for the Earth,* and if you haven't yet seen the film or read the book, Al Gore's *An Inconvenient Truth* is a must.

- There are plenty of green magazines and science journals in different countries, as well as online newsletters and websites like *www. greenpeace.org, www.RMI.org* (the website for the Rocky Mountain Institute), *www.sierraclub.org, www.rachel.org* and many, many more.

- Finally, we recommend Bill Bryson's bestselling *A Short History of Nearly Everything.* A comprehensive and entertaining history of science, it contains cautionary tales that will improve your critical overview of technology; it also confirms the narrowness of the margin in which human life exists.

Sustainability starts with your own body

What we eat and how much exercise we get play a major part in the health of our planet. In simple economic terms, society faces 'guns or butter' choices between spending its resources in areas like preventing global warming, or in propping up health systems collapsing under the weight of inactivity, poor eating habits and stress. The burgeoning trillions of dollars being spent on the latter is money which we literally do not have available to spend on more important things. We *must* learn to look after ourselves better: to exercise daily, eat food that is healthier for our bodies and the planet, and reduce our stress levels.

The strategies and techniques described in Parts One and Two of this book will help you to achieve healthy, sustainable exercise and eating habits. Employers need to help with this, for example by providing shower and locker facilities, and healthy food in their cafeterias. Governments also need to help, especially in the area of school curricula. There has been research around for years showing that children achieve more, not only physically but also academically, when given vigorous daily exercise, yet education systems the world over have dramatically reduced PE in recent decades! If you're a parent, push for more PE at your kids' schools and insist that they serve healthy, organic wholefoods in their cafeterias instead of junk.

When it comes to stress, we pointed out in Part One that fitness and strong social relationships are the best remedies, and we also talked about the synergistic power of exercising with your friends and family. In addition to this, try some relaxing activities like meditation and massage; have a few sessions with a skilled counsellor or life coach; laugh a lot; read great books and go to the movies; stay in one place and put down deep community roots; make as many friends as you can and spend plenty of time with them. Research has shown that this last point alone can prolong your life by more than ten years.

Conduct environmental audits of your home and workplace

This is a rapidly growing field of business. These days, any architect, construction company or energy provider has connections with local experts, or just Google 'environmental audit' or 'energy audit' to find advisers in your area. In New Zealand, try the Energy Management Association (*www.ema.org.nz*). The California Energy Commission's Consumer Energy

Center — *www.consumerenergycenter.org* — is a good website for do-it-yourself information and links. The website *www.greenhomeguide.com* is another good site with information and links to various US suppliers. Prepare yourself to ask expert questions by reading relevant chapters of *Natural Capitalism*, one of the books recommended at the beginning of this chapter.

The following are some recommendations that an environmental auditor is likely to make:

• Switch to a green energy supplier, or to a green option offered by your existing supplier.

• Solarise your hot water supply using simple, inexpensive technology. After an initial payback period, this will mean a saving of 40–70 per cent of your energy bill! Modern installation techniques enable this to double up as a source of winter heating.

• Completely solarise your house or business with solar cells. Most energy companies offer the option of drawing energy from the grid when you need it, and selling your excess electricity back when you don't. If your supplier doesn't do this, then switch companies. The Whispergen systems discussed in Chapter 9 are another extremely efficient and low-cost source of energy.

• Insulate your home. Insulating your ceilings and walls and under your floors, blanketing your water heater, sealing off draughts, double-glazing windows etc will dramatically reduce your heating bills.

• Switch to CFLs (compact fluorescent light bulbs) or the even more efficient new LEDs (light-emitting diodes). CFLs use a quarter of the energy of standard bulbs and last years longer. LEDs are new technology and currently need special installation, but they use almost no energy.

• Turn off unused lights and appliances. More than 30 per

cent of electricity consumed in homes and offices is standby power used to keep appliances running in the 'off' position.

● Next time you replace an appliance, purchase one with a high energy-efficiency rating. Some of the newer systems use a fraction of the energy of older ones. If your old machines still have a way to go, don't feel guilty about this: it takes energy to produce new things, so conservation has its value too. But wash clothes and dishes only when you have a full load, select cold- or warm-wash cycles over hot ones (better still, turn down the temperature on your water heater), let your dishes air-dry and hang your clothes out in the sun (aside from saving energy it's a much more effective germ-killer than the dryer).

● Conserve water, even if there is currently no water supply problem in your area. It takes a huge amount of energy to pump in water then pump away wastes. Fit low-flow showerheads and toilet systems. If your toilet isn't ready to be replaced, then the old brick-in-the-cistern trick works wonders. You'll be amazed at how much you'll save on your water bill.

● For even bigger savings and smaller environmental impacts, install a water tank on your property to collect rain, and water your garden via gravity feed rather than a pump.

● Have your pipes checked for leaks by an expert. A 2007 report on municipal water losses in London stated that the city was losing billions of litres of water a year through aged, leaking pipes.

● Eliminate as much waste as possible by recycling and composting.

● Use natural ventilation by installing floor vents and opening windows in the summer rather than running an air-conditioning system. This saves a huge amount of energy and avoids the bacterial nasties that accumulate in AC refrigeration units and ducting systems.

The principle we mentioned earlier applies here. You don't have to do everything at once, just do what you can afford, bit by bit, as quickly as you can. Of course if you're constructing a new house or building, for an additional cost of three to five per cent you can install the latest technology. You will save yourself many times that amount in the long term and add dramatically to the value of your asset; in New Zealand, green buildings achieve valuations of around 30 per cent more than traditionally constructed ones.

Green your mode of transportation

As we stated in Chapter 3, around 20 per cent of CO_2 emissions in developed countries come from cars. Commercial trucking accounts for another 13 per cent. Imagine the wonderful effect on the planet if, over the next decade, we all switched to hybrid cars; better still, to shared or public transport; or, best of all, to walking and riding bikes. The health effects of the last option can be dramatic.

Experts believe that to ensure the survival of human civilisation past the mid-21st century, we have to reduce our CO_2 emissions by 70–80 per cent over the next few decades, maybe sooner. We can save a substantial part of that by changing our transport habits.

Companies have a responsibility to help in this. They can assist employees to work from home for a few days each week, and encourage the use of public transport, carpooling and walking and cycling to work. Some might even consider introducing incentives for employees to live close to their workplace.

One of the world's biggest companies, Wal-Mart, has become a poster child for green business, saving itself an estimated US$300 million per year in the process of becoming eco-friendly — greening its buildings, reducing packaging, designing better systems etc. At the transport end, Wal-Mart has saved tens of millions by introducing low-friction tyres to its trucking fleets (and keeping them fully inflated), reforming transport routes and keeping engines correctly tuned.

Why not become an advocate for green business yourself? You'll slash long-term costs and your staff and customers will love you for it.

Governments also have to help. The US freeway systems that allow multi-passenger vehicles and hybrids to use special lanes are a good start. Building great public transport systems is even better. Top of the list is creating safe bicycle pathways that encourage people to ride bikes without having to risk their lives in city traffic. Yes, these things are expensive and will take years to achieve — all the more reason to get started right away.

When Phillip's father became mayor of Auckland, he opened the books to discover half a billion dollars worth of deferred maintenance on water and sewage systems — a significant amount in a city of this size. Nobody had dared to touch the problem because of its magnitude, but a simple plan in which the work was carried out bit by bit over a number of years made it manageable.

The world needs more politicians with the vision and commitment to act long term. Why not join a local environmental lobby group yourself, or stand for election to a local council? You'll be taking on a long-haul fight, but you can make a difference.

It may not be popular to think so, but we believe that significant fuel taxes are essential, along with other taxes that will make clear the true costs to society of various industrial activities. If these taxes are not introduced, Victorian technologies will stay in place, blocking the advent of clean, sustainable alternatives that are available right now. It's taken 50 years to cut cigarette smoking in half. Education and publicity were important, but the most successful countries were those that made it the most expensive. With global warming, we do not have 50 years to wait.

Fifty final recommendations

We've left the last word here to our researcher and colleague, career environmentalist Richard Tong. The box on pages 271–278 contains his 50 recommendations — philosophical, political and practical — for preserving this wonderful planet.

In reading these, or any, environmental recommendations, it's important to realise that research around most of the subjects in this book is evolving day by day. At one time we would have said that one of the most important things you could do was to plant as many trees as possible — completely reforesting the planet as a way of soaking up CO_2. However, research has been published stating that trees in temperate zones may actually soak up heat and slightly increase global warming, and that we should be focusing on planting them only in tropical zones. With more research, these findings might be contradicted again. But certain types of trees and other vegetation are still likely to be net global warming inhibitors, even in temperate zones, during their growth phase (after which it remains necessary to keep them as carbon storage sumps, as opposed to clearing them, which results in the release of their carbon).

Trees have many other benefits, of course, such as preventing erosion and pollution, and creating sanctuaries for wildlife — birds, for example, which in turn support other parts of our ecosystem through pollination, seed dispersal and insect and rodent control. So we'll await with interest the development of research in this area. In the meantime, we recommend giving as much support as possible to charitable organisations involved in defending tropical rainforests. You can find many of these by Googling 'rainforest protection'. Only two per cent of the rainforests remaining on earth have formal protection. Many voluntary organisations have been set up to help safeguard the remaining 98 per cent. These include:

- Conservation International *www.conservation.org*
- Fauna & Flora International *www.fauna-flora.org*
- Friends of the Earth *www.foe.org*
- Forest Stewardship Council *www.fscoax.org*
- Global Forest Watch *www.globalforestwatch.org*
- Greenpeace International *www.greenpeace.org*
- IUCN — The World Conservation Union *www.iucn.org*
- Native Forest Network *www.nfn.org.au*
- Rainforest Action Network *www.ran.org*
- Rainforest Alliance *www.rainforest-alliance.org*
- Rainforest Foundation UK *www.rainforestfoundationuk.org*

- Rainforest Information Centre *www.forests.org/ric*
- Rainforest Rescue *www.arborday.org*
- Tourism Concern *www.tourismconcern.org.uk*
- World Rainforest Movement *www.wrm.org.uy*
- World Wide Fund for Nature *www.wwf.org*

Similarly, environmentalists have argued against air travel. However, there's recently been a subtle shift. In *The Weathermakers*, Tim Flannery points to evidence that the negative effects of aircraft may be outweighed by their complex contribution to global dimming, a phenomenon presently countering some of the effects of global warming. Again, we'll await new research in this area with interest.

Thankfully, along with the evolving research there are new solutions cropping up continually. To see the environment becoming a major political issue in countries around the world has been both remarkable and inspirational. It seems that every day the media report some ingenious new idea or venture aimed at making a positive contribution. We are confident that the current challenges will bring out the best in us; that the human race will display its most noble and inspirational traits in rising to, and ultimately overcoming, these most dire threats. This will not be easy, but that's all the more reason to get started now. We'll say it again: Those of us who can, must.

● RICHARD'S 50 RECOMMENDATIONS

1. Remind yourself and others around you that each and every individual is important. Remember that the Red Cross was founded by one person, Henri Dunant. More prosaically, in Walt Disney's words: 'It all began with one little mouse.'

2. Encourage mandatory courses in philosophy, ethics and environmental studies at all educational levels. Consider doing some more courses yourself.

3. Reflect on the four cardinal virtues of all the major religious traditions in an environmental context: prudence, justice, temperance and fortitude. Are we allocating resources in a just way? Is it prudent to fill the atmosphere with greenhouse gases? Are we being temperate when we extract and use every last drop of oil? How are we going to find the fortitude to deal with some of these issues?

4. Encourage friends and family to think seriously about family planning. Each child in over-developed countries like the United States or New Zealand places a disproportionately large burden on the Earth in terms of energy and resource use.

5. Do not think that it is a new thing for humans to hit resource limits: this has been going on for millennia. The only difference now is that we have global reach and there are no useful new frontier lands to conquer. As a result, we have to think smart. That is not difficult, but we have to face up to it and make sure that we are not just replacing one problem with another.

6. Find out where your food and water come from, and where your refuse and sewage go, and push for the highest levels of waste reduction, recycling and treatment.

7. Be on the lookout for, and stay wary of, any politician or business claiming to have a quick or high-tech fix for an environmental problem. Such solutions probably won't work; even if they do, they are only going to fix one thing and quite possibly make others worse. Some of the extravagant claims for genetic engineering fall into this category, likewise some of the moves towards palm oil or ethanol as replacements for oil as a fuel; each brings its own environmental problems.

The prospect of a massive development of nuclear energy in its present form to solve energy, and security of energy supply, problems is more likely to create a nightmare scenario with few of the claimed benefits. You need fossil fuels to make the concrete for the massive installation and fossil fuels to mine the uranium. Ever heard of a terrorist attacking a wind farm or targeting an experimental tidal power station?

8. Make a regular donation of money to an environmental group and/or low-technology development agency. The regularity allows the group to plan and budget. Keep an eye on the activities of your chosen group(s).

9. Stay in one place and put down deep community roots. Join a local environmental lobby group or consider standing for election to a local council. Anticipate the need for stamina but do not assume that you do not have a contribution to make.

10. Make submissions to the statutory planning agencies for your community. Ask yourself if corporate or council strategic plans have any element of 'strategy' or are they just wish lists. If they are wishy-washy, say so.

11. Worry less about issues of left and right (e.g. public versus private ownership), because both tend to avoid the issues on the main environmental agenda (designing waste and pollution out of the system and developing equitable resource allocation).

12. Support transparency in government at all levels. We have to have transparent donations to party machines and registers of lobbying by business and interest groups. Everyone is entitled to be involved, but secrecy is not in the public interest.

13. Promote the provision of serious facilities for cyclists and pedestrians. For too long, footpaths and cycleways have been afterthoughts tacked on to the edge of roads, at best; it is time, instead, to marginalise cars and trucks. Try suggesting covered and walled routes for bikes and pedestrians to offer a comfortable and safe experience for those who are prepared to put their own energy into moving around. Let the cars get jammed up: more drivers will convert to cycling and walking.

14. Drive less and support public transport. Try video conferencing. Investigate working from home for one or two days a week.

15. Push for goods to be sent by rail and sea, not road and air. Promote tolls and other charges for road-using vehicles. Require that road is not favoured over rail in terms of taxes and subsidies.

16. Lobby for serious green design so that products have minimal to zero impact throughout their manufacture and entire life cycle. Many products, like cars and computers, use more energy in their manufacture than during their use. It is important to know which ones are efficiently made, as well as the ones that are efficient to run. Check out the green labelling systems that operate in your area.

17. Call for serious resource accounting so that balance sheets for all businesses include environmental impacts. At the moment, everyone has to complete financial reports for taxation and shareholder reporting purposes. We need to promote triple-bottom-line reporting, whereby environmental and social performance are measured and reported on annually as well as finance.

18. Demand environmental auditing as a mandatory requirement — with minimum standards for existing operations. Many new business operations on new sites have to meet strict environmental regulations that their competitors avoid through being well established.

19. Ask yourself which individuals in history you most admire. Many people choose giants like Jesus Christ, Mahatma Gandhi, Mother Teresa or Nelson Mandela. Reflect on why they are so different from our contemporary celebrities.

20. Plant a vegetable garden or grow a few plants in pots. Teach a child to raise seeds and plants. Too many children have no idea where their food comes from. Try to persuade schools to involve children in gardening and tree planting on a regular basis.

21. Travel by plane as little as possible, but if you do go overseas try to visit one or more of the less developed countries and get a feeling for the pressures they are under.

22. Set yourself a serious carbon charge. Put aside, say, 50 per cent of all expenditure on fossil fuels, petrol, gas, airline tickets etc. Use the money to fit a solar water heater and examine other solar initiatives. If family or friends have holiday houses, encourage them to go solar.

23. Go to *www.consumerenergycenter.org* and do a simple energy audit. Check what your own energy supplier offers, because it might be more suited to your local conditions. Remember to implement the suggested changes.

24. Plant two long-lived trees that are native to your area each year. Seek expert advice and select trees that prefer a warmer climate zone and plant in a location where you can be reasonably certain that they will be secure. If you have difficulties finding a site, ask your local council.

25. If you or your relatives are farmers, plant trees or encourage them to do the same. Based on New Zealand evidence, up to 30 per cent of the land area can be planted in trees without reducing pastoral productivity.

26. Pave as little of your land as possible and save rainwater for gardening, toilet flushing and clothes washing.

27. Consider installing water-saving features in your household even if you live in an area with no major water supply problems.

28. Take civil defence seriously. We can expect more extreme weather events and every bit of planning pays dividends. Make sure you know about people in your neighbourhood who might need help.

29. Learn the weed and pest species in your locality and assist in removal/eradication programmes.

30. Remind someone that sustainability and carbon neutrality are both very good ideas but difficult to achieve. Remind yourself that aiming for sustainability is not instinctive. Try writing a sustainable business plan.

31. Read some of the serious green authors, especially Schumacher, Commoner, Suzuki, Diamond, Monbiot or Flannery (as detailed earlier in this chapter). Do not waste time reading popular apologists for the 'business as usual' approach or writers picking a hole in one specific environmental issue. They are missing the point, which is the sum of all the issues.

32. Forget any ideas of gaining short-term advantage in the marketplace from being 'green'.

33. Make a point of meeting some of 'they', as in: 'They'll come up with something.' Ask yourself if you are really happy to have your future in 'their' hands.

34. Ask how your community compares to others in terms of water and air quality. You might be surprised, as there are very few industrial cities that shape up well.

35. Encourage innovation by workmates, employees etc. It is possible to design and implement low-impact solutions, often very cheaply.

36. Criticise all your own environmental actions and invite criticism from others. In that way, you retain control. Inviting and accepting criticism is the only way to achieve excellence and we need some serious, honest excellence to deal with the more intractable problems.

37. Learn the meaning of some original local placenames;

sometimes they reveal important historical facts about the environment in the area.

38. Take photographs of landscapes, environmental features, heritage places or plants that are important to you, date them and file them away. It is amazing how poor one's memory can be in situations where things change slowly. Photos are the best way to show how much sand has been lost or gained, or how much the landscape has changed etc.

39. Sort out your own environmental priorities and be honest about them. Using 'environmental' arguments, like concerns about visual pollution to criticise environmentally sound initiatives such as a wind farm, may hide a personal agenda.

40. Try to develop the ability to look at things from a pessimistic point of view yet deal with them optimistically. In other words, be prepared for the worst yet be happy to tackle the job with hope.

41. Demand that your legislators introduce mandatory deposits for containers because reusable container systems save vast amounts of energy and waste.

42. Pressure your legislators to introduce mandatory deposits for consumer durable items like cars, computers and whiteware. Very often these pieces of equipment have hazardous components and the people who built them know best what is in them and how to safely recycle them.

43. Give your used furniture and clothing to charity outlets for reuse by others. An enormous amount of energy goes into the manufacture and supply of goods and giving them a longer life ensures better use of the embedded energy in each item.

44. Learn to read the ingredients on food packages and avoid those that have a huge array of preservatives, additives and colourings. Check out the various organic food products available in your area and find one or two that you trust.

45. Buy and eat fresh, locally grown, organic produce. Get to know your growers and give them feedback about what you do, and do not, like. Do not expect your organic vegetables to last as well as conventional produce because they have not been chemically treated to stop the natural process of sprouting.

46. Cut down on the amount of meat and fish in your diet. Try vegetarian or vegan meals and support good vegetarian and vegan restaurants; they provide an introduction to high-quality fresh vegetarian food for many people.

47. Demand that your supplies of meat are grass-fed and free of hormones and antibiotics. Do not purchase irradiated food. Buy only certified free-range eggs and double-check the producer's claims.

48. Ensure that the local businesses you support with your hard-earned money are following your lead. Ask if they have a recycling programme or compost their food wastes. Do they have a champion for environmental initiatives in the firm?

Write letters or send emails to any organisation involved in something you feel uneasy about and tell them. Send a copy to your relevant elected official. The main reason they have not given the environment a higher priority is because not enough of us have told them to.

49. Push for absolute transparency in decision-making at every level of corporate and civil governance. It is not acceptable to hide knowledge about environmental impacts or health effects behind commercial or governmental sensitivity.

50. Develop ways to restrict the influence of the professional lobbyists who now represent an enormous force against adapting to the changing world. They represent corporate dinosaurs who do not want to change.

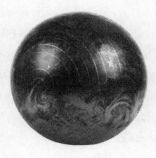

acknowledgements

In writing this book we drew on the contributions of many people. We'd like in particular to acknowledge the work of Auckland journalist Simon Farrell-Green, Les Mills writer Sacha Coburn and Auckland environmental scientist and author Richard Tong, who all passionately believe in the cause and have given us huge amounts of help and guidance. We cannot find words to adequately express our gratitude to you three. Our deepest appreciation also goes to Russell Hill of Les Mills, and the many others who gave advice and input to the final script.

To Nicola Legat from Random House New Zealand — thanks for your undying patience and support: we could never have done it without you.

Rebecca Jones ND, managing partner at Jackie's clinic, the Holistic Medical Centre in Point Chevalier, Auckland, is responsible for much of the medical research incorporated into Chapter 7. Rebecca, along with Dr Helen Smith MD, runs a medical practice that is unique in the world.

Thanks to Joanna McMillan-Price, author of the Les Mills BodyRevolution nutritional guides, from which we sourced some of the material in Chapter 5.

Thanks to Nic Hall and Jeremy Taine for the book cover and for your contributions to internal design.

Our profound thanks to all of the Les Mills New Zealand and Les Mills International (LMI) teams who run those remarkable organisations and who have all played a part in developing the systems we talk about in this book — in particular, Jill Tattersall, CEO of LMI, without whose brilliance and dedication that company would have achieved only a fraction of what it has. Thanks also to LMI's national agents and all the inspirational fitness-industry leaders who work with them, and in particular to Bill Robertson, at Les Mills Asia Pacific, who played a huge part in getting LMI off the ground.

Thanks to John McCarthy, former president of the International Health, Racquet and Sportsclub Association (IHRSA), for two decades of inspiration, and to IHRSA itself for its excellent health research information service. Thanks also to the members of our fitness industry roundtable group, in particular to Will Phillips, our convener.

We are deeply indebted to those who have given us guidance and help over the years, in particular Brian Kreft, Marco Marinkovich, Denham Shale, Gerard Curry, Jill Tattersall, Barbara Blakey, and our fathers, Les Mills and Peter Bull.

Finally, thanks to our family and friends who support us and make our lives so much fun.

Here's to the future!

Phillip and Jackie

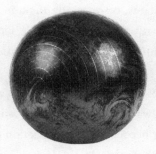

a note about numbers and references

Waiheke Island is an idyllic spot in Auckland's Hauraki Gulf just 30 minutes by ferry from the centre of town. It has a resident population of about 7000, which swells to 45,000 in the height of summer. In June 2005, an idiot wrote to the Prime Minister claiming to have witnessed the release of material contaminated by foot and mouth disease on farms on Waiheke. Because New Zealand is a major exporter of agricultural produce we take biosecurity issues very seriously and officials swung into gear immediately. From their records they expected to find 34 farms on the island; in fact, they found 99 farms and 57 of these had animals on them. It is not often that anyone gets to do an absolute census of anything and check it against the written record; when this happens and there is a significant gap between the record and reality it is very sobering. In this case, official records were nearly 300 per cent out.

Throughout this book we have tracked down verifiable facts and figures, but there will always be another figure for, say, the amount of fish caught or the water consumed in America. Choose any one fact and search the internet for it — for example total world rice production — and look at ten different websites that turn up; you will find figures that vary wildly. In some cases they are defining 'rice' differently ('paddy rice' is a greater figure than 'milled rice') and in others they are mixing up the units. American tons (or short tons) are 2000 lbs or 909 kg; British tons (or Imperial or long tons) are 2240 lbs or 1018 kg; and metric tons or tonnes are 1000 kg. Often it is impossible to know whether figures from different countries are measuring the same things. Does a total for domestic waste in New Zealand represent the same sort of refuse as in the United States, or does one include some commercial waste or litter because traditionally that's how it's collected? In other cases figures may be manipulated intentionally, as in some statistics for the tonnage of fish caught.

Noting these traps does not imply that the facts are in doubt, but it does mean that someone will always be able to produce a different number. In most cases this does not matter because it is the direction of the underlying trends which is critical. If the disease claim on Waiheke Island had been true and not a hoax, the precise number of farms would likely have become a relatively minor issue because local knowledge would have tracked them down anyway. Similarly, whether the world runs out of oil in 30, 40 or 50 years' time is probably not worth arguing about, when it is the combustion products of that oil that are threatening us.

appendix 1

Weight-loss tips checklist

Start with the simplest and work your way through. Set yourself a target date to complete at least 12 items on this list and cross them off as you go.

☐ **Cut junk food from your weekly shopping**
If it's not in the cupboards you can't eat it

☐ **Cut out soft drinks and sodas**
They are pure poison — discover the wonderful taste of water

☐ **Stop buying fruit juice**
Eat fruit instead

☐ **Skip the snacks**
Start eating three correctly sized meals a day

☐ **Start serving smaller portions**
Gluttony is one of the seven deadly sins for a reason; it's never attractive

☐ **Stop preparing multi-course meals**
Start a one-plate-per-person per meal habit

☐ **Learn to make a great salad**
In fact, learn to make ten great salads

☐ **When eating out, just order an appetiser**
A small resolution, but every bit helps

☐ **Start buying healthy snacks for your kids**
Carrots can be cool

☐ **Start making healthy food fun**
Teach your family to love all the good foods

☐ **Learn to make a great soup**
A subtle change to your diet, a huge change for your health

☐ **Drink water**
Lots and often

☐ **Institute a balanced-plate system**
Smart carbs, power-packed proteins and healthy fats with loads of veges

☐ **Switch to low-fat food options**
But be careful of the low fat/high sugar trap

☐ **Have coffee, fast food and alcohol wisely and in moderation**
Don't be sucked in by the 'supersize' scam

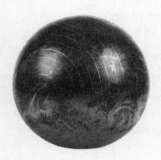

appendix 2

BodyTrainer energy levels

WOMEN		MEN	
Weight (kg)	**Energy Level**	**Weight (kg)**	**Energy Level**
< 60	1	< 80	7
60–69	2	80–89	8
70–79	3	90–99	9
80–89	4	100–109	10
90–100	5	110–120	11
> 100	6	> 120	12

Bodytrainer food group daily blocks

Energy level	Group 1 Vegetables	Fruits	Group 2 Carbohydrate - rich foods	Group 3 Protein –rich foods	Group 4 Fat –rich foods	Group 5 Occasional foods
1	> 5	2	3	4	2	Optional— swap one carbohydrate block and one fat block
2	> 5	2	4	4–5	2	
3	> 5	2	5	5	3	
4	> 5	2	6	6	3	
5	> 5	3	7	7	3	
6	> 5	3	8	8	4	
7	> 5	3	8–9	8–9	4	
8	> 5	3	9	9	4	
9	> 5	4	10	10	5	
10	> 5	4	10–11	10–11	5	
11	> 5	4	11	11	6	
12	> 5	4	12	12	6	

Bodytrainer food group daily blocks

Please note that the recommended food blocks here are based on the recommended energy intake targets for people with average daily activity levels (see page 243). You may need to adjust these if you are an extremely active person. If you are in that category, however, you'll be in such great shape that you probably won't need the techniques given in this chapter!

© Les Mills International 2002

GROUP 1 VEGETABLES — UNRESTRICTED

Aim to make vegetables the biggest portion of the meal and always include in both main and light meals — the greater variety, the better. Approximately half a cup of vegetables equals one block. Options include:

Asian greens	Asparagus	Bean sprouts
Beetroot*	Broccoli	Brussels sprouts
Cabbage	Capsicum/peppers	Carrots*
Cauliflower	Celery	Courgette/zucchini
Cucumber	Eggplant/aubergine	Endive
Fennel	Green beans	Kale
Leeks	Lettuce	Mushrooms
Onions	Parsnips	Peas
Pumpkin*	Radishes	Rocket
Spinach	Spring onions	Squash*
Tomatoes	Turnips	Watercress

* Marginal

FRUIT

One block equals:

Medium-sized fruit

1 apple	1 banana	1 nectarine
1 orange	1 peach	1 pear
1 persimmon		

Smaller fruit

2 apricots	1 cup berries	2/3 cup cherries
½ cup grapes	2 kiwifruit	2 plums
2 tangerines		

Other fruit

½ cup of fruit salad   ½ cup canned fruit   ½ cup stewed fruit

½ grapefruit   ½ mango   1 cup diced melon

1 cup diced pineapple

Dried Fruit

6 dried apricot halves   4 dried dates or prunes   2 dried figs

1 tbsp sultanas, raisins or currants

GROUP 2 CARBOHYDRATE-RICH FOODS

Your smart choices are those with a low GI, indicated by ☺. Choose these on most occasions.

BREADS	**ONE BLOCK EQUALS**
Bagel	½ bagel
Crispbreads	2 sandwich size/4 small
Crumpet	1
English muffin	1
Flour tortilla ☺	1 medium
Heavy fruit loaf	1 slice
Pita bread ☺	½ medium
Pumpernickel bread	1 slice
Scone	1 small/½ large
Sourdough bread ☺	1 slice
White or wholemeal bread	1 slice
Whole-grain bread ☺	1 slice

BREAKFAST CEREALS	
All-Bran varieties ☺	¾ cup
Breakfast biscuits	2
High-fibre flake varieties	1 cup
Natural muesli ☺	½ cup
Oatmeal ☺	¼ cup
Porridge ☺	1 cup cooked
Rolled oats ☺	⅓ cup

GRAINS

Asian noodles ☺	½ cup cooked, ¼ cup dried
Barley	½ cup cooked, ¼ cup raw
Brown, basmati/Koshihikari/Doongara rice ☺	½ cup cooked, 1/6 cup raw
Bulgur wheat ☺	½ cup cooked, ¼ cup raw
Couscous	1 cup cooked, ¼ cup raw
Pasta ☺	½ cup cooked, ¼ cup dried
Polenta	1 cup cooked, ¼ cup raw

STARCHY VEGETABLES

Bean or lentil-based soup ☺	½ cup
Beans or chickpeas	¾ cup cooked, ¼ cup dried
Lentils ☺	¾ cup cooked, ¼ cup dried
Potato	1 fist-sized, 3 small/new
Sweet potato ☺	1 fist-sized, 1 cup mashed

SNACK FOODS

Low-fat cereal bars	1 x 40 g bar
Muesli bar (choose <10 g fat/100g)	1 x 30 g bar
Pretzels	30 g packet
Rice cakes	3
Rice crackers	15 small crackers

GROUP 3 PROTEIN-RICH FOODS

MEAT, FISH & POULTRY	**TWO BLOCKS EQUAL:**
Fish	100 g raw, 75 g cooked
Mussels/oysters/other shellfish/prawns	½ dozen, 50 g cooked
Red meat or game	100 g raw, 75 g cooked

SEAFOOD	**ONE BLOCK EQUALS:**
Canned fish	½ small can, 40 g
Eggs	2 medium-sized
Sardines	3 small fish
Sliced cold meat	2 slices, 40 g
Smoked salmon	50 g

DAIRY AND SOY ALTERNATIVES | **ONE BLOCK EQUALS:**

Cottage cheese	3 tbsp, 50 g
Light soy drink	1 cup
Low-fat milk or flavoured milk	1 cup
Low-fat yoghurt	½ cup, 150 g carton
Reduced-fat cheese	30g, ¼ cup grated, 1½ slices
Tofu	½ cup, 130 g

LEGUMES (AS PART OF VEGETARIAN MEAL)

Beans or chickpeas	¾ cup cooked, ¼ cup dried
Lentils	¾ cup cooked, ¼ cup dried
Bean or lentil-based soup	1½ cups

GROUP 4 FAT-RICH FOODS

ONE BLOCK EQUALS:

Avocado	¼ fruit, 1 tbsp mashed
Butter, margarine	2 tsp, 10 g, 1 individual pack
Hummus	¼ cup, 3 tbsp
Nuts and seeds	2 tbsp, 20 g, small handful
Oils	½ tbsp
Peanut butter	3 tbsp
Tahini (sesame butter)	3 tbsp

GROUP 5 OCCASIONAL FOODS

DEDUCT ONE CARB & ONE FAT BLOCK:

Carrot or banana cake	Small slice, 40 g
Chocolate cookies/biscuits	1
Chocolate, milk or plain	4 squares, 28 g bar
Commercial burger in a bun	½ serve
Crisps/chips	1 x 25 g packet
Fancy cake	¼ slice
Hot chips/fries	10 chunky, small handful fries
Ice cream	2 rounded scoops
Plain biscuits	2

ALCOHOLIC DRINKS

Beer	1 can/bottle, 375 ml
Light beer (reduced alcohol)	2 cans/bottles
Spirits	2 x 30 ml nips
Wine	1 glass, 150 ml

FAT-TREE TREATS

DEDUCT ONE CARB BLOCK:

Fat-free confectionery, sweets/candy, jellies	25 g or small handful
Low-fat desserts	individual carton or small serve
Low-fat ice cream	2 scoops

Healthy calorie intake for safe weight loss: energy levels table

| Level | Weight (kg) | Targeted energy intake | | Targeted daily macronutrient intake | | |
		Kilojoules	Calories	Carbohydrate (g)	Protein (g)	Fat (g)
Women						
1	50–60	5000	1200	130–145	60–80	35–40
2	60–70	6000	1400	160–175	75–95	40–45
3	70–80	6500	1550	170–190	80–100	45–50
4	80–90	7000	1650	185–205	90–110	50–55
5	90–100	7500	1800	200–220	95–115	50–60
6	>100	8000	1900	210–235	100–125	55–65
Men						
7	70–80	8500	2000	225–250	105–130	55–70
8	80–90	9000	2150	240–265	115–140	60–75
9	90–100	10000	2400	265–295	125–155	65–80
10	110–110	10500	2500	280–310	130–165	70–85
11	110–120	11000	2650	290–325	140–170	75–90
12	>120	12000	2850	320–350	150–185	80–95

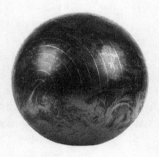

index